MINDFULNESS

& STUTTERING

Using Eastern Strategies to Speak
with Greater Ease

ELLEN-MARIE SILVERMAN, PH.D.

ISBN: 1478385111
ISBN 13: 9781478385110

Library of Congress Control Number: 2012914455
CreateSpace, North Charleston, SC

Other Books by Ellen-Marie Silverman

Jason's Secret

Mind Matters. Setting the Stage for Satisfying Clinical Service. A Personal Essay

Contents

1   WHAT YOU NEED TO KNOW BEFORE READING ON   1

2   HOW MINDFULNESS HELPS   13

3   MINDFULNESS   21

4   MINDFULNESS MEDITATION   29

5   TWO MINDFULNESS MEDITATION PRACTICES   49
    FOR STUTTERING

6   FOUR ADDITIONAL MINDFULNESS PRACTICES TO   79
    PROMOTE CHANGE

7   CHANGING   113

SUBJECT INDEX   131

REFERENCES   137

RESOURCES   153

ACKNOWLEDGMENTS   157

ABOUT THE AUTHOR   159

1

WHAT YOU NEED TO KNOW BEFORE READING ON

When Vice President of the United States Joseph Biden (2009) received the American Speech-Language-Hearing Association's Annie Glenn Award for his inspirational efforts to overcome his stuttering problem, he reminded us that the work involves commitment, perseverance, and curiosity. Those of us with stuttering problems know this to be true. We recognize that to speak as we wish requires whole-heartedly doing what is required for as long as it takes while remaining open to what change brings. For me that was mindfulness.

MINDFULNESS PRACTICE

I began practicing mindfulness in 1996 to enrich a waning meditation practice begun in 1973 to better manage stress *shenpa*

(Silverman, 2009c). Fortunately, I had no expectation, or even suspicion, that mindfulness would help me address my stuttering problem which had resided silently beneath the surface of my life for decades until it re-emerged in 1980. If I had, knowing as little about the process of mindfulness practice as I did and being as impatient as I was, I probably would have quit a few days later when I failed to observe any change in the way I approached life or how I communicated. I enjoyed practice as a break from work and family responsibilities that I believed would somehow make me happier, more peaceful, and more pleasant to be around. But when I encountered a then little-known mindfulness-based practice of working with *shenpa* (Chödrön, 2003a) following a prolonged and fierce re-emergence of stuttering, I saw it as a potent tool. As a speech-language pathologist, I immediately realized that the practice, like no other I knew, could help me and others like me speak more as we wished by skillfully addressing habitual thoughts and behaviors arising from feeling ill-at-ease (Silverman, 2005). *Shenpa* work, I decided, was capable of helping release those of us from stuttering problems the fear of speaking sparked and stoked.

MINDFULNESS, SHENPA, AND STUTTERING

Shenpa is a Tibetan word referring both to our discomforting urge to react to what we dislike in ways that we know increase unpleasantness for us and our difficulty refraining from doing so (Chödrön, 2005; 2003a). Making sarcastic comments to people who irritate us is one such example. Self-medicating with comfort food, drinking, taking recreational drugs, or engaging in compulsive sexual practices when we are anxious or when things fail to go as we wish are others. When I encountered an article by Pema Chödrön (2003a) describing *shenpa* as a root of unhappiness, I recognized that stuttering problems could be likened to *shenpa.* From what I had been told and from what I remember about speaking when I was three and began stuttering, I believed my problem stemmed from resisting stuttering, as does many people's. So, I hypothesized that working skillfully with *shenpa* could help offset stuttering problems (Silverman, 2005).

Fortunately, since *shenpa* work depends upon the application of mindfulness, I already had been practicing mindfulness meditation since 1996 using the ancient Buddhist techniques of *shamatha-vipassana,* or calming and focusing the mind, sometimes referred to as insight meditation (e.g., Kabat-Zinn, 2005; Silverman, 2009c; 2009b; 2005; 2003). So, I layered *shenpa* work, which emphasized staying rather than fleeing strong emotions and sensations, onto my existing mindfulness meditation practice. The combined practice helped me remain present rather than drift into reveries reliving unpleasant encounters or spin fantasies about my future whenever I felt challenged by speaking.

Staying with the fear of stuttering provided the space to make specific, helpful accommodations to communicate as I wished even as I stuttered, something I had not done before. Eventually, by adopting the Buddhist practices of *maitri,* or unconditional positive self-regard (e.g., Boorstein, 2008; Salzberg, 2005), to relate kindly to myself at all times and *tonglen* (e.g., Chödrön, 2003b) to recognize I am more alike than different from others and by silently reciting short poems called *gathas* (e.g., Hanh, 2006) and proverbs from *lojong* mind training (e.g., Chödrön, 2007) to reinforce my intent to be mindful, I established the combined practice that has helped me satisfactorily address my stuttering problem.

In the chapters to follow, beginning with the next and concluding with the last, I describe these practices and their application to stuttering problems, and I identify means of addressing obstacles to implementing them in whole or in part. I share my knowledge and experience as an individual who has had a stuttering problem and as a clinical and research speech-language pathologist with the intent of revealing actual and potential benefits associated with practicing mindfulness meditation not to provide a tutorial about stuttering problems, *per se.* Numerous textbooks (e.g., Guitar, 2005; Williams, 2004; Conture, 2000;), novels (e.g., Beckwith, 2008; Fusco, 2004; Silverman, 2001), scientific and professional journals, and websites offer information about stuttering (Please see the Resources section). I believe that the reader of this book, a person with a stuttering problem, someone interested in learning about help for people with stuttering problems, a professional, or a student-in-training would possess some knowledge about stuttering problems and would be looking primarily for help deciding whether practicing mindfulness meditation would provide a useful role in learning to speak with greater ease. Therefore, this book addresses the practicality and usefulness of applying the ancient yet contemporaneous Eastern self-care practice of mindfulness meditation to stuttering problems, (e.g., Silverman, 2009; 2005; 2003) while incidentally referring to features of stuttering problems many people experience.

MINDFULNESS AS A SECULAR ACTIVITY

Do not be concerned: You do not need to be Buddhist to apply the methods I describe. These tools have been and are used by people of various religious affiliations and people with no religious affiliation at all (e.g., Boyce, 2010; Ponlop, 2010; Kabat-Zinn, 2005; Keating, 2002; Boorstein, 1998). *Shamatha-vipassana, shenpa, tonglen, lojong, maitri,* and the use of *gathas,* associated with East-Asian, particularly Tibetan, Buddhism, which collectively comprise the protocol I developed for my personal use, described in Chapters 5 and 6, can be undertaken as purely secular activities. By applying them, we no more become Buddhist than we become Jewish when we follow directives from the Jewish Scriptures to love our neighbor as our self (Leviticus

19:18) or to refrain from coveting (Exodus 20:13). Rather than drawing us away from our customary religious and spiritual affiliation or non-affiliation, mindfulness meditation seems to enrich our particular transpersonal outlook. For instance, Father Thomas Keating, Trappist monk and Abbot of St. Joseph's Abbey sought instruction from the Zen Buddhist Master *Roshi* Sasaki prior to co-founding the practice of Christian contemplative prayer, Centering Prayer, and its derivative, Welcoming Prayer (e.g., Keating, 2002). Jews (e.g., Kamentez, 2007; Boorstein, 1998) have found deepening fulfillment practicing Judaism while maintaining Buddhist-based mindfulness meditation practices. And some find that these tools encourage an appreciation of life seemingly separate from circumscribed faith-based or spiritual beliefs (e.g., Kabat-Zinn, 2005). If these accounts fail to dispel your concern that using Buddhist-based mindfulness meditation tools may draw you from your present religious and/or spiritual path, then you may want to put aside these practices for now. As always, trust your instincts.

STARTING A MINDFULNESS PRACTICE TO ADDRESS STUTTERING

Intellectually, you may want to dismiss the idea that an adult can find relief from a long-standing stuttering problem by applying yet another change protocol. That is understandable if you have participated in years of therapy and experimentation or if you believe stuttering problems are genetic in origin (e.g., Kang, et al., 2010). But the only way you actually will *know* whether mindfulness may help you find greater ease speaking is by trying this ancient, non-invasive, low-cost method that contemporary research in the United States and elsewhere reveals modifies not only adults' beliefs and behavior but also the structure and organization of their brains (e.g., Baime,

2011; Schwartz and Gladding, 2011; Siegel, 2010a; Begley, 2007; Davidson & Harrington, 2001). Perhaps, mindfulness will help you change as you wish. Perhaps, it will not. Experiment thoughtfully. Be patient. Changes associated with mindfulness occur in their own way and on their own time-table. They can not be forced any more than the ripening of ears of corn can be hastened by tugging on the plant's roots. But, with sufficient exposure to conditions that nourish, such as rain, sunshine, and a temperate climate and adequate protection from damaging conditions, such as hail, parasites, and hungry raccoons, they flourish. And with nourishment and care so, too, can our efforts to live mindfully, especially when infused with curiosity, courage, and enthusiasm. And as Vice President Biden suggested, and as some of us know, taking responsibility for desired change does not mean needing to go it alone. If you think mindfulness can help you or if you think it can not, you might benefit from consulting the resources listed at the back of this book.

Please recognize this slim book as a presentation of a coordinated, integrated practice, or *schemata,* of specific mindfulness meditation practices I personally have combined to satisfactorily address my stuttering. As such, it is a book *about* meditation, not an instruction manual *in* meditation. For those drawn to the idea of practicing mindfulness meditation, books, CD's, DVD's, magazines, websites, and podcasts provide information and demonstrations. Face-to-face guidance from trained teachers can be found at established centers, such as The Insight Meditation Society in Massachusetts and The Spirit Rock Meditation Center in California, where the practices of *shamatha-vipassana*, or mindfulness meditation, and *mairtri* are taught. Representatives from each site may be able to suggest resources near you for more accessible instruction and guided practice. Please refer to the Resources Section of this book.

Being Pragmatic

Deciding whether or not meditating may help without experiencing meditation may lead to an unwarranted conclusion. We might presume meditation is too passive to satisfactorily address the robust features of our stuttering problem, because we believe that meditating is just sitting still. Meditation often takes the form of sitting still. But the experience of sitting still in meditation is a dynamic one in which we learn skillful ways of working with thoughts, emotions, and bodily sensations as they arise. That is why meditation often is referred to as *practice.* What we learn sitting we apply to the rest of our life (e.g., Boyce, 2011; Loori, 2008). Only by meditating can we know whether the practice will provide more of what we need to know to change as we wish (Kongtrül, 2006), just as we can not know what it is like to have a stuttering problem without actually having one, even if we deliberately stutter in public or over the telephone. Genuine experience makes the difference.

If meditating appeals to you as a means to help you live life more as you wish, then make a commitment to do the work. And be curious, thoughtful, persistent, and patient doing so. Andrew Weil, M.D., (1995) believes it takes eight weeks, or approximately two months, to start noticing the effects of actions undertaken to generate functional change in the body, such as lowering blood pressure, increasing energy and a sense of well-being, improving physical and mental endurance, loosing weight, and so on, a time frame recently corroborated in neuroscience studies investigating the effect of mindfulness on brain structure and function (e.g., Baime, 2011). While some effects of *shamatha- vipassana*, or mindfulness meditation, can be experienced during the first session, transferring that experience to every day life takes some time. So we can not expect the practices described in this book to be usefully applied to stuttering for some time after beginning them. How long that will be I can not say, nor, I believe, can anyone else. But what I can say is that, with daily practice supplemented by learning about building a mediation practice from teachers such as Pema Chödrön (e.g., 2005; 2004b; 2003a), Thich Nhat Hanh (e.g., 2009; 2003), Jack Kornfield (e.g., 2005), Sakyong Mipham (e.g., 2007; 2006), Sylvia Boorstein (e.g., 2008), Sharon Salzberg (e.g., 2011; 2006), and Joseph Goldstein, (e.g., 2006), whose teachings are widely available, and through personal consultations with trusted teachers, you should know within several months whether, through meditating, the quality of your life is improving as you intend. If it is, then your effectiveness applying mindfulness to stuttering also should be increasing. You can talk about this with an experienced meditation teacher and, perhaps, with a speech-language pathologist as well.

If, for whatever reason you choose not to begin meditating or quit, then you have made a discovery of what does not seem to be useful for you at the present. Congratulate yourself! You are now better informed about yourself than you were. And that is what considering or trying new methods of change is really about. Keep exploring to find what meets your needs and what does not seem to. Consider carefully why in each instance, and you will be learning a great deal about yourself you will find useful living life as you wish. As you know, just because some method or methods do not seem to have helped you as you wish does not mean you can not become as you wish. All that means is that you have not done so yet. As the famed inventor, Thomas Edison said when he experienced disappointment after disappointment experimenting with the construction of the filament that would turn the electric light bulb from a dream into a reality, *"Well, I haven't failed; I've found 1000 ways that don't work."* Like he, we come closer to achieving what we wish only by thoughtfully working to do so.

As you may surmise, reading about applying mindfulness practices to stuttering problems may invite you to view stuttering problems and treatment for them in somewhat unfamiliar ways. If you do not allow this to discourage you from carefully considering the concepts introduced, this slight reframing may, of itself, help initiate desired change. We all know, but sometimes forget, that to become as we wish, we need to adjust what we believe to change what we do. As Albert Einstein bluntly advised, *"Doing the same thing over and over and expecting different results is the definition of insanity."* If we think the same, we will do the same. If our goal is to communicate differently, we benefit from changing how we conceive of ourselves and the world, for *"When we change the way we look at things, the things we look at change* (Dyer, 2009)" for good or for ill. Such is the power of a new point-of-view.

Positive Ripple Effects from Practice

The assertion has been made and alluded to several times that to experience the effects of mindfulness on stuttering requires practicing mindfulness. This seems obvious but needs reflection since some, inexperienced with the practice, may consider it no different from simply "paying attention" and decide all they need to do to apply mindfulness to stuttering is to pay more attention to their stuttering, a plan that not only may fail to help them speak with greater ease but may suggest mindfulness will not work for them and may not help others. Anyone who has practiced mindfulness even once, as the meditation teacher Pema Chödrön (2005) wryly comments, knows how challenging it is. The key instructions, "Get comfortable. Relax. Watch your breath. If your attention wanders, return it to your breath" seem easy to follow. But, when you try to apply them, you, too, quickly will discover just how difficult it is. That is why what is embodied in mindfulness can helpfully address matters associated with our stuttering only after first learning how to be mindful. Initially, that may be only during meditation sessions, which is the reason they are called *practice.* Later, when certain skills, such as returning to following the breath after noticing we are talking to ourselves in our head, become stabilized, we apply them to other aspects of life that are more challenging than sitting, such as waiting in line at the convenience store, being stuck in traffic, or waiting for the furnace to be repaired. That is when the effects of practice begin to permeate how we live by softening, then dispersing, limiting beliefs and practices. And that is when we can begin to apply what we are learning about being mindful to our stuttering problems.

FOR THOSE WHO HELP

If, by chance, you happen to be a therapist wondering whether the practice of mindfulness can help a client overcome a stuttering problem, this book also may help you decide. While the presentation focuses on adults' stuttering problems, mindfulness has potential for application to children's stuttering problems as well, since children can successfully practice mindfulness for self-help purposes (e.g., Greenland, 2010; Willard, 2010; Hanh, 2011b; 2010a; 2006; Greco & Hayes, 2008). One suggestion: Before you offer counsel to adult clients or to parents about practicing mindfulness, incorporate mindfulness into a segment of your own life if you are not already doing so, perhaps, through conscious eating (e.g., Kabat-Zinn, 2005), mindful cooking (e.g. Brown, 2010), mindful shopping (e.g., Goleman, 2010) or some other everyday activity. When you personally experience what is involved practicing mindfulness, you will be able to empathically as well as intellectually appreciate the cost-benefit ratio involved to help guide you to make the useful recommendations your clients may request (e.g., Geller & Greenberg, 2012;   Siegel, 2010b).

A REASONABLE EXPECTATION

Living mindfully brings a sense of self-mastery that comes from learning to quiet and strengthen our mind to see more clearly and to act more skillfully. No longer tossed about by fearful thoughts that generate strong emotions we have not yet learned to skillfully manage leading us to behave in ways we sometimes later regret, we can learn to communicate with greater ease by using the tools we are learning in meditation practice to live mindfully. Doing so, we become increasingly self-confident. We live and speak with greater ease. We have changed.

2

HOW MINDFULNESS HELPS

MINDFULNESS AND NEUROPLASTICITY

Perhaps, you have heard: Practicing mindfulness reduces stress and improves the quality of life (e.g., Boyce, 2011; Kabat-Zinn, 2005). If so, you may be wondering whether practicing mindfulness may help you find relief from a stuttering problem or remove the remnants of a once bothersome one. Your questioning may have led you to do some reading about mindfulness and to talk with some people who knew some people who practice mindfulness, and you are unsure. You realize that, while you may feel refreshed, even more energetic, if you live mindfully, you question how attending to the way you live can resolve a robust, long-lived stuttering problem. After all, like others, you may have watched your stuttering and watched for your stuttering to wage war against it for years without noticeable benefit. In fact, you may recognize that your vigilance actually worsened your problem by heightening your anxiety. But, as you also may surmise, mindfulness, as a specific practice, differs appreciably from apprehensive watching.

Being mindful, we calmly observe what we are thinking and doing and what is going on in and around us. We note our thoughts, emotions, and bodily sensations as they arise as well as the sights, sounds, smells and other sensory stimuli impinging upon us from outside. And we do not judge. We simply observe. And that relaxed manner of non-judgmental observation has an enormous upside. Recent research findings inform us that mindfulness not only helps us focus to be more as we wish but modifies our brain so we become increasingly so (e.g., Siegel, 2010a; Begley, 2005; Mayberg, *et al.*, 2002; Davidson & Harrington, 2001). This striking discovery regarding the adult brain's *neuroplasticity,* defined as its ability to reorganize itself to acquire new skills, legitimizes therapy. Neuroplasticity, it seems, depends on calm, focused attention. It also leads us to modify the adage, *"When we change the way we look at things, the things we look at change,"* to *"When we change the way we look at things, what sees the things we look at changes."* But the first requirement is to look at what is inside and outside of us. If we do not do that carefully, it is unlikely we will change to be as we wish no matter how many books and articles we read, how many therapists and healers we ask for help, how many instruments we buy, or how many nutritional supplements and pharmaceuticals we ingest. It is up to us to first look at our lives and how we live them if we want to experience life differently.

You may be intrigued that mindfulness, a non-invasive, low-cost, primarily self-directed practice, can lead to profound and lasting change, but you also may be apprehensive about using it as a self-help tool if you know that some mediation teachers discourage doing so as distracting to mindfulness practice itself. Yet, doing so is what other meditation teachers recommend (e.g., Hanh, 2009; Mipham, 2006; Chödrön, 2005). They remind us that the Buddha introduced mindfulness practice more than 2,600 years ago to relieve suffering. That is why these teachers encourage using mindfulness, which can be a secular practice (e.g., Kabat-Zinn, 2005; Keating, 2002; Boorstein, 1998), as it has been for me, to improve personal and work relationships and to increase health and happiness and they teach how to do that (e.g., Mipham, 2006).

BEYOND REASON ALONE

The Age of Reason ushered in by Descartes and other philosophers in the 17th Century encouraged many of us to believe we can resolve personal problems with rational thought. But thought alone rarely succeeds in bringing desired change, especially if our goal is to alter established behavior patterns. Several years ago, I painfully remembered this is so. I learned that a prominent teacher of mindfulness advised students to breathe deeply to experience a calm, clear mind. Greater mental clarity was a goal I had set for myself, so, given his stature, I embraced his advice. I recognized my habitual breathing pattern was shallow, and I tended to stutter when frightened or excited, occasions when I was breathing even more shallowly. Having taught university courses on the anatomy and physiology of the speech mechanism and on disorders of the speaking voice to speech-language pathology majors, I realized breathing diaphragmatically would help. It would at least increase the oxygenation of my blood. But I was busy and did not want to add more tasks to my daily schedule so I easily convinced myself I did not need to practice. I told myself I knew how to breathe deeply and could apply the technique when I felt strong emotion cloud my thinking. Such is the power of rationalization. As a clinician, I knew substituting a new, competing behavior pattern for an established one required considerable practice of the new pattern to create motor pathways strong enough to be dominant, especially under stress. So, a few weeks after deciding to implement deep breathing when needed, I predictably failed to do so the first time my resolve was tested. While waiting for a local anesthetic to take effect prior to a root canal procedure, I was hyperventilating and sweating and experienced one of the longest and most involved blocks of my life (Silverman, 2006b). Had I been practicing abdominal breathing, it may well have been my habitual pattern, and I would not have needed to remember to utilize it. I would have been doing so, and I may have been calm and mindful enough to stutter more easily, if at all, rather than stutter as I did. And I may have been less damp!

Rationalists like to believe we can reason our way out of problems. If we can envision a solution, we can achieve it. But, as empiricists and everyone who has tried to alter established behavior patterns, such as a golf swing, the fingering of a musical chord on a guitar, or the quality of speech, knows, desired change may start with an idea, but materializes through thoughtful, consistent effort. Only skillful, committed practice can develop new, desired behavior patterns with the strength and resiliency to substitute for established, competing ones under stress. There is no other way to get where we want to be without skillful practice. And skill-building practices occasionally can be boring, uncomfortable, frustrating, and, even, frightening when we encounter aspects of ourselves we would rather keep invisible. Mindfulness meditation practice is no exception. Sitting erect on a cushion or chair to meditate for 10, 15, or 20 minutes at a time when we are tired or achy; stressed from work, family, and social commitments; bored with the quintessential task of managing our wandering mind; or daunted by facing feelings of anger and sadness that can arise during meditation provides challenges to be met with endurance, patience, and no small amount of kindness. As Jack Kornfield (1993), psychologist and teacher of mindfulness meditation, suggests, learning to meditate is like training a puppy to stay. When it strays, we gently bring it back and once again tell it to stay. We do this over and over until the puppy learns to stay. And, just as with training a puppy, we can not know how long it will take to train our mind to be present enough to allow us to work satisfactorily with our stuttering.

Had I begun meditating to find relief from stuttering, I doubt I would have realized the communication benefits I have. Impatient by nature I would have ditched the practice shortly after I began it. I did not know then that the benefits of practice emerge slowly, seemingly imperceptibly at times, following an order and a time timetable all their own. That this is so and that it is not work for " . . . the faint hearted" is now generally known (e.g., Kabat-Zinn, 2005). So, the only way to actually know for yourself whether mindfulness may provide the change you seek is to doggedly practice for several months free of expectation other than that of a more settled, focused mind. If you have accomplished that and you find meditation congenial, then you may find mindfulness helpful in working with your stuttering problem.

Knowing what we are thinking and doing in the moment is crucial to changing as we wish. We realize that. But, until we learn the power of mindfulness to bring us more fully into the present and help us stay, we may think simply saying *Pay Attention!* to ourselves or using some other such commonplace reminder to be mindful provides direction enough. At least, that is probably what many of us wish who prefer quick solutions to challenges. Yet, by the time the final *n* of *Pay Attention!* fades, our minds already may be drifting from one memory to another, from one apprehension to another. Just as teaching a horse to accept a rider requires an informed plan, sound equipment, and repetition, so, too, does teaching our minds to be present and stay present. Acquiring the skill of mindfulness to speak more as we wish requires qualified instruction and practice that we fortify through endurance and patience.

A PROCESS

Mindfulness, attending calmly, without judgment, to what we are thinking, feeling, and doing, strongly contributes to reducing or eliminating our stuttering problems, since the opportunity to change exists only in the moment. The more mindful we become by attending to *what is* rather than anticipating what might be or regretting what was, the more capable we become of creating the change we want. We can not stutter differently in the past. We can not be certain we will speak differently in the future. The only time we actually can influence how we speak is in the present. And what we think and what we do there moves us into circumstances we desire, or not. It has been said: *"The past is history. The future is a mystery. Now is a gift. That's why it's called The Present."* The present is our power point. And mindfulness gets us there and helps us stay. What we do then makes all the difference.

How do I know mindfulness effectively addresses stuttering? From my personal experience as someone who has practiced mindfulness for 16 years, has worked as a clinical and a research speech-language pathologist, and has a stuttering problem. As do others with stuttering problems (e.g., Bloodstein, 1969), I recognized long ago I mentally disengaged from my immediate surroundings before I needed to speak or believed I might. I fled at Mach IV speed to where I could indulge a whirlpool of thought about the need to make a good impression and the possible consequences if I did not. When my awareness snapped back to the launching pad of my hasty departure, sensing, perhaps, a need to represent self-interest, I re-entered the scene slightly confused and somewhat embarrassed because I grasped the superficialities of the immediate circumstance but few of its subtleties. I was uncertain how to correctly relate. So, what did I do? I decided whether or not I needed to speak. If I thought I did, within a nanosecond or so, I was gone to worry once again about the impression I might make. Such was my fear of speaking incorrectly.

I also was not present when I stuttered. When I repeated a word or felt I was strangling from a tight, prolonged vocal fold stoppage, I silently launched the lament of many newly oppressed, "*Why is this happening?*" Still repeating or breathless and wide-eyed bemoaning my unwanted, fiendish predicament, I became slightly more proactive. I mutely cursed the stuttering, which, of course, did nothing to dismiss it. Finally, my need to change what I was doing took more practical form. I pulled and yanked and pushed and shoved to wrest myself free of the errant behavior of my body. Eventually, I was speaking as I usually did and concluded my reactions had worked. So, the next time I stuttered, I repeated the routine. Every time I did, I was no more aware of my surroundings than when I feared I might need to speak. I did not attend closely to what people said or how they said it and what they might really be saying and wanting. I did not monitor my posture or bearing. I directed my attention to forcing myself back to speaking as usual.

I was hardly there, wherever there was, if speaking was a possibility or if I stuttered. So, much of my life, I was engrossed in resisting what might be or what was or fearing my imagined future. I did not need to practice mindfulness to learn that. I had known that most of my adult life. But, by practicing mindfulness meditation, I learned I could be present even when stuttering and, by doing so, I could more readily speak and communicate as I wished. I also learned that, basically, I am the same as everyone else. It seems the Buddha, who introduced the method 2,600 years ago or so, recognized that most of us rarely are present whether we stutter or not. We all seek what we think will make us happy and flee from what we think will not and, in doing so, fail to experience lasting satisfaction. So, we often become frustrated, even discouraged. But we do not have to live like that. We can learn to be present even when we feel uncomfortable, such as when we stutter. Mindfulness can help us do that to communicate more satisfactorily.

3

MINDFULNESS

Sometimes to understand what something is, we first need to consider what it is not. To more readily appreciate the benefits of cultivating mindfulness, we begin by briefly reflecting on a common state of often risky and generally stultifying functioning referred to as *mindlessness*. We can then appreciate the help we receive addressing our stuttering problems by cultivating the relaxed awareness to know what is happening inside and outside ourselves in the moment, pleasant and unpleasant, which is called *mindfulness*.

MINDLESSNESS

Absent-Minded. Distracted. Forgetful.

All three serve as descriptors of mindlessness. Perhaps, you remember a day when you arrived at work without your bag lunch. You thoughtfully assembled it. You placed it on the kitchen counter where you usually do. But, leaving home thinking about the deadlines you needed to meet that day, you absent-mindedly failed to pick it up and take it with you. Or, maybe, like so many, you have driven to your home, a hardware store, or some other location without being able to recall what you passed along the way because recalling in detail a recent argument with your partner, thinking about paying the bills, or wondering whether to buy or lease a new car distracted you from the task of driving. And, perhaps, you may have found yourself standing in the family room at home without remembering how you got there or why. These common experiences exemplify *mindlessness*, a foggy state of mind in which we fail to be fully aware of the circumstances of the moment. We are functioning mindlessly when we distract ourselves from the present with regret, worry, fantasy, planning, or denial to avoid directly addressing what we consider the boring, common-place, and fearful inside and outside of ourselves.

For many of us, mindlessness is a well-known state of being. We wake with a fever surprised to find ourselves ill because we believed we were well when we went to bed the night before. Then we recall our experience of unexplained body aches and pains and extreme fatigue that we pushed through the previous two days. We did not want to slow down. We did not want to recognize our body as unwell. We wanted to do what we had planned, so we chose to live in mindlessness until we could no longer ignore our body's acute need for special care. Had we been mindful of its earlier messages by resting, drinking more water, and increasing our intake of healing substances, such as Vitamin C, we might not be so ill this day as to require several days to heal.

Similarly, we sometimes seem astounded to be stuttering. Repeating words or parts of words, unable to release our voice, bobbing or jerking our heads about, and so forth can take us by surprise as the tension we had been accumulating in our bodies erupts in a burst of stuttering. We had noticed the tension build-ing moments earlier and had responded in our customary way of suspecting we might stutter and vowing or hoping we would not. When we realized we were stuttering, we tried to quickly push through and past the stutter or conceal it, and probably stuttered longer and more forcefully while generating disturbing facial and bodily mannerisms that have become part of our stuttering *gestalt* or stopped speaking before we said all we wanted to say. If, instead, we had responded to the sense of tension increasing in our facial, neck, laryngeal, and thoracic musculature by relaxing into rather than combating it, we might have stuttered much less noticeably, if at all. (*Relaxing into stuttering* is a technique discussed in the *shenpa* section of Chapter 5,"Two Mindfulness Practices for Stuttering.")

Risky and Stultifying

We recognize mindless living as risky. We see how behaving absent-mindedly, distracted, and in forgetfulness can set us up for mishaps, large and small, physical and social, as we seek to avoid facing the prickly, challenging, or mundane circumstances of the moment to experience pleasantries and amusement instead. But what we do not so readily see is that mindlessness generates a stultifying climate basically unfavorable to creating desired change. Functioning mindlessly, we are not alert enough to our thoughts and behavior as they occur to make timely corrective changes to be more as we wish. Instead, we can find ourselves in a waterfall of distracting thought distancing us from what actually is happening (Kornfield, 1996). For example, we unexpectedly may recall stuttering in high school gym class choosing sides for volleyball practice, then on a critical job interview, then when meeting future in-laws, then when ordering a deep dish pizza at the new take-out pizzeria, and so on, one such reverie morphing into another, leaving us only marginally connected to the present. All the while we fondly, angrily, or sadly reminisce, we easily can loose sight of the fact we may be holding our breath and tensing our thoracic, laryngeal, neck, and facial musculature. This mindlessness renders us temporarily unable to apply techniques we believe can help us speak with greater ease then and there. An easily run-away, distracted mind, the type almost all of us have almost all of the time whether we have a stuttering problem or not (e.g., Hanh, 2003), shackles us to behavior we no longer wish to continue. That is why we need to be as mindful as we can to change as we wish.

MINDFULNESS

Breathing in, I know I am breathing in.
Breathing out, I know I am breathing out.

- - - (Hanh, 2006, p. 32)

This *gatha,* one of many short verses associated with southeast Asian Zen Buddhism, helps set our intention to be mindful, and, as such, helps define mindfulness. (See the *gathas* section of Chapter 6, "Four Mindfulness Practices to Promote Change".) Being mindful, we know how we wish to function, and we know how we *are* functioning (e.g., Langer, 1990). We know what we are doing. We know when we are feeling uncomfortable or pleasant sensations in our body. We know when we are experiencing emotion. And we know when we are thinking. We can know this each moment. And, each moment, we also can know what is happening outside our bodies. We notice exhaust fumes from gas-powered motors, emissions from faulty gas furnaces, scents from lilac and rose blooms, smoke from barbeques, odor from soiled diapers, and so on. We attend to emergency sirens, dogs barking, thunder rolling, arguments, referee whistles, and so forth. We witness people pushing grocery carts down the sidewalk filled with their personal belongings, the full moon, traffic slowing down ahead of us, leaves beginning to fall from trees, flames rising from the roof of an adjacent apartment house, and the like. We notice the temperature and the humidity. And we rely on our senses to decide whether or not we are somewhere safe. Being mindful, we notice what is inside and outside our bodies and decide whether and how best to act to be free of danger and to be happy.

What we discover we accept without judgment. We do not reject what is because it scares us or disgusts us or saddens us. We recognize what is simply as information. Observing rain, for instance, we can respond by deciding to stay indoors until it stops, being grateful the earth is receiving needed moisture, making paper boats to float down the gutter when the rain stops, checking whether the sump pump is working, or doing all, some, or none of these. Whether we like that it is raining or not makes no difference. It *is* raining. Resisting that reality because we feel angry, sad, or scared will not stop the rain from falling, but it may forestall our moving forward. Accepting what is, we can grab an umbrella as we leave for our medical appointment or a magazine to hold over our head; we do not cancel our meeting with the specialist

You may be wondering, *What does all this have to do with stuttering?* I believe more than we may know. When we recognize what we are thinking and doing in the moment and accept that as what is without excitement or aversion, we can then, and only then, take the constructive action we need to communicate as we wish then and there. We only can change in the moment, not in the past or, even, in the future. As Ekhart Tolle (2005) reminds us, the only place we can change is *The Now*. As we do so increasingly, we do so with ever greater ease.

Intentional, Relaxed Awareness

As expressed in Chapter 1, being mindful, we choose to calmly observe what is going on inside and outside of us (e.g., Siegel,

2010a). We do not search for a particular thought or a specific behavior to arise, we simply notice what is. Like a thermostat set to maintain room temperature to our satisfaction, we pre-select how we wish to respond to our thoughts and behavior and then do so with unwavering focus. That is our intent. Putting it into practice, like implementing other ideas for desired change, is not easy. In fact, it can become quite frustrating. Jon Kabat-Zinn (2005), founder of mindfulness based stress reduction (MBSR) counsels that being mindful is ". . . *not for the faint-hearted.*" Observing our attention wander and accustomed, unhelpful behavior reemerge, we calmly and patiently redirect our attention and behavior to what we wish them to be, time and time again.

We refrain from self-abasement when we lapse. And we do not entertain feelings of regret or discouragement. We recognize reverting to past behavior as inevitable when learning new, competing behavior and resume our mindfulness practice without attendant feelings of recrimination or remorse or fantasies of inevitable and lasting failure. We return to our practice with kindness toward ourselves. We are, after all, doing what we believe is best for us. Sometimes we experience joy, even awe. We feel grateful, special, relieved. We consider the experience as a sign that finally we are doing it right. We long to re-experience that bliss. We tell ourselves anything else is failure. By talking to ourselves that way, we set the stage for being discouraged and, possibly, quitting. Sometimes we will feel good about our ability to attend to what is happening, and sometimes we will not as our mind seems speedy. Eventually, we learn that a good experience meditating is relating skillfully to what is. It is not the experience we have that informs us as to whether or not we are being mindful but the manner in which we relate to what we experience. Learning to be mindful without attachment to the outcome of being mindful, we become increasingly present wherever we are. How we do this is the subject of Chapters 5 through 7. For now, what matters is to recognize that, as a sign in a gambling casino proclaims, "You have to be present to win." (Kornfield, 1996). So it is with gambling, and so it is with living our lives.

ATTENTION AND FOCUS IN EVERY-DAY LIFE

How broadly and carefully we observe what we do and experience depends upon what we deeply believe. I recall when I was so terrified of making a bad impression by talking that I scarcely heard what others had to say during conversations. Now, listening at least as much to others' words as my own, I speak when I believe doing so will be helpful. Free of constraints I previously imposed on myself by believing conversing was all about how I performed releases me to appreciate the give-and-take of friendly and even heated exchanges. Attending to the larger purpose of an encounter to appreciate the opportunity to be useful as well as the chance to strive for personal and collective goals enriches our knowledge base and elevates our social skills. Viewing our role primarily as speaking without making a mistake accomplishes neither. This is what attention and focus contributes to mindfulness.

What we believe about ourselves, others, and the world around us establishes our sphere and focus of attention and, ulti-mately, our satisfaction with being (e.g., Silverman, 2009a). As Albert Einstein reminded us, "We live what we believe. "

4

MINDFULNESS MEDITATION

Before I began mindfulness meditation in 1996, thoughts streamed through my mind distracting me from what I was doing, especially from routine activities, such as eating, brushing my teeth, washing my hands, bathing, and so forth. I moved through life like most, mindful only a moment or so every now and then (Mipham, 2006). That became astonishingly clear when I took a six-week, Level 1, *hatha yoga* class in 1980 to deal more effectively with the stress I was experiencing at work and at home. Rather than performing exercises mindlessly while keeping count of the number of times I repeated them as I was accustomed to doing in other classes, here the focus was on observing and utilizing our mind-body interplay as we gently entered, held, and exited *asanas*, or specific postures. The instructor directed us to observe our body and our breath and co-ordinate the two. Directing my body to perform as he instructed was doable and enjoyable, but monitoring my breath while holding postures was challenging. Thoughts distracted me, mentally pulling and pushing me here and there. My actual experience of viewing mind-body interplay was occasional and fleeting. It seems this slow-paced, deliberate activity unmasked the torrent of almost moment-to-moment mental activity my usual, frenetic life accommodated.

Gradually, I learned to focus on manipulating my body into unfamiliar positions and calmly maintaining them using breath to help. Before the final class, I decided to take the Level II class, but the instructor would not let me. He said, somewhat harshly, that my mind was too noisy and that I needed to repeat Level 1. I was stunned. I was proud of what I had learned experientially about the interplay of my mind and body. I felt ready to learn more. And I did not take negative judgments of what I did easily. Lacking the knowledge and experience to appreciate the deeper meaning of what he was telling me and driven by self-righteous anger, I decided to continue practice on my own, which I did for many years thereafter bolstered by what I learned from watching yoga programs on public television and video tapes. And, in time, I came to realize how helpful the instructor's message was. By learning to quiet and steady my mind, eventually with the help of *shamatha-vipassana*, I became more peaceful and better able to work skillfully with my mind and body together to make adjustments on-the-spot to increasingly speak and live in a manner I wished (Silverman, 2009b; 2005; 2003).

THREE FUNDAMENTAL BENEFITS

Using *shamatha-vipassana* to strengthen and hone my ability to be mindful led to three fundamental changes in my outlook and behavior that has helped me be more as I wish in any circumstance and at any time. They are: Less Negative Self-Talk, Greater Self-Mastery, and Greater Openness. The one with the most wide-reaching influence is the reduction in negative self talk. Eliminating doubtful and critical thoughts about what I would experience and what I could do about it by staying open to what life brings and learning to be confident in my ability to make sound decisions and follow through with them led to a sense of greater self-mastery with a companion willingness to be more open. An increasing ability to be mindful helped fashioned them all.

Less Negative Self-Talk

Teachers of mindfulness meditation refer to the steady stream of self-talk we all produce almost all the time as a waterfall of thought (e.g., Kornfield, 1996). It is as though we have a built-in analyst that compulsively comments on what we experience through a continuous out-pouring of messages that can distract us from life around us (e.g., Tolle, 2005). But we are not doomed to information overload or living in our heads. We posses a tool we can use to disable this often useless and sometimes harmful accessory. And that tool is mindfulness. When we monitor our thoughts, we can chose to act on those that require our attention and release those that do not, such as chronic, repetitive warnings of possible present and future difficulty speaking and the relentless remembrance of unpleasant experiences of stuttering.

By being mindful, which allows us to be attentive and discerning, we can become more calm and focused and chose to act in ways that help us change as we wish (e.g., Kornfield, 1996). But by yielding, as we usually do, to such negative self-talk, we can immerse ourselves in a climate of fear of stuttering that provokes habitual mindless reactions obstructive rather than supportive of desired change in the moment (e.g., Silverman, 2008).

You may wish to observe the waterfall for yourself by simply sitting quietly where you are not likely to be interrupted by outside events.

Select a chair, preferably non-upholstered, and sit near the edge of the seat so that your spine is erect but not rigid. Get comfortable. Relax. Then instruct yourself to listen to the sounds inside the room for 10 minutes. If you are like many with no formal meditation experience, you will find yourself drawn almost immediately instead to regrets, fantasies, plans, and worries big and small. By the time you end the experiment, you probably will have realized you were thinking almost the entire time you were sitting. You may have heard the radiator hissing as it released steam and a toilet running and nothing else because you entertained a thought that led to another, and another, and another tumbling after and mixing with one another.

That jumble of thoughts is the waterfall. Learning to respond skillfully to it in meditation practice readies us to be more focused and sharp doing what we know helps us speak more as we wish

Increased Self-Mastery

It has been stated that the greatest form of mastery is self-mastery (Mipham, 2006). That is no less true about stuttering. We speak with greater ease by working to master our thoughts about and our responses to our stuttering. We do not need to master our stuttering to speak with greater ease; we need to master ourselves (Silverman, 2011).

For me, the most unsettling aspect of stuttering has been the sense of losing control of my body. Not guilt. Not shame. Not embarrassment. But fear. When I was a child, I believed my unplanned, unwanted repetition of words and syllables and abrupt, forceful speech stoppages signified I was being attacked by an outside force or forces, and my body was failing, possibly dying. Even as an adult, I reacted by struggling fiercely against stuttering as if I were in a life or death battle with some outside force.

But rarely did I emerge feeling entirely free. I surfaced haunted by the clammy fear I would be tracked down yet again and would need to wage yet another tough fight somewhere, sometime. To minimize the possibility, I spoke as little as possible, a not uncommon decision among people with stuttering problems and one that generates troublesome consequences of its own (e.g., Silverman, 2006a; 2003; Silverman and Williams, 1968).

Mindfulness meditation provided the perfect antidote to those unhelpful beliefs and behaviors, although I did not realize it at first. I began the practice in 1996 to better manage stress. Then, quite serendipitously, seven years later, I encountered the practice of working with *shenpa,* which involves remaining and working with rather than fleeing and resisting what seems disagreeable (e.g., Chödrön, 2003a). Incorporating that practice into my evolving *shamatha- vipassana* meditation practice of calmly and generously observing my thoughts, sensations, and behaviors during everyday life was transforming. I realized *My Stuttering Is Me!* Stuttering is not a phantom throttling me. Stuttering is not a villainous adversary stalking me. Stuttering is not a poltergeist taunting me. Stuttering is not an *It* of any sort. *Stuttering is what I do.* I stutter, and I resist stuttering. And, when I fight with my stuttering, I am fighting with myself. That enshrines my stuttering problem, which is an idea I first encountered as a graduate student at The University of Iowa. I even shared its message with clients. But, until I applied the techniques of mindful self-observation and the tools for redirecting and calming my mind mindfulness meditation teaches, I failed to experience the fullness of its truth and to satisfactorily put it into practice: *I make my own stuttering problems. If I want to overcome these problems, I need to think and act differently.* Mindfulness helps.

I have no more knowledge of why I or anyone else stutters than I ever have, but I know that by committing to conquering stuttering we become a house divided. To free ourselves from the inevitable frustration created by engaging in such a winless contest like a dog chasing its tail requires a different approach (e.g., Carroll, 2010; Allione, 2008). We decide to become master of the house. We create the climate and set the tone. We keep it in good repair. We appreciate the shelter it provides. And we calmly address whatever needs our attention on our own or with the help of capable individuals who possess knowledge and skills we have not yet acquired. We rest in the knowledge we are in charge but not alone.

Greater Openness

> *". . . I live my life in widening circles*
> *that reach out across the world. . ."*
> - - - Ranier Maria Rilke (Barrows & Macy, p. 45)

As we develop and use mindfulness to become more accustomed to recognizing our thoughts, being with our emotions, noticing our bodily sensations, and monitoring our actions as they arise and more skillful relating to them, we become more participatory (e.g., Hopkins, 2008). Our increasing self-mastery brings greater confidence in our ability to relate along with the desire to live life more fully. We listen more carefully and fully to others, no longer fiercely distracted by worrying whether we will stutter. We are more willing to speak-up at home, with acquaintances, with strangers, and even with those we consider difficult. And we become more willing to speak in diverse settings. We even feel more kindly toward others, having begun to relate more kindly to ourselves, which mindfulness meditation encourages. We recognize and appreciate our undeniable kinship with and responsibility toward all others and cease to feel separate. Knowing we are not alone, we experience more joy. Our walk is lighter, our smile more at the ready, our energy more plentiful, and our speech more pleasurable. We have begun to heal.

FOUR CORE FOCUSES OF PRACTICE

Four core focuses of mindfulness meditation practice individually and collectively provide rich soil for personal change, including the forms considered the three fundamental benefits. These practices are: Calming the Mind, Looking and Seeing, Staying with Emotions and Sensations, and Experiencing a Sense of Ease. Although I present each separately, in practice they intersect and co-mingle as they do in everyday life the way the facets of a jewel reflect each other to magnify its brilliance. For instance, Looking and Seeing frequently involves Staying with Emotions and Sensations, and Looking and Seeing and Staying with Emotions and Sensations leads to Experiencing a Sense of Ease while Calming the Mind forms the foundation for these practices. Keeping that in mind, let us consider each singly.

Calming the Mind: Shamatha

As I became aware during *hatha yoga* classes, minds can generate an unending stream of distracting thought diminishing our opportunity to function fully in the moment. We are so accustomed to this ongoing mental chatter we barely recognize it until we become still. Then we see how it can drag us into reveries or push us into fantasies, distancing us from the present, the only place and time where we possess power to change (e.g., Kabat-Zinn, 2005). Some refer to this restless and relentless mental activity as *Monkey Mind* because it resembles a monkey jumping about and chattering. But we can quiet and focus our run-about mind through mindfulness meditation so that it becomes a tool that serves us well. Training our mind, we begin to see what actually is before us. We learn to recognize thoughts, emotions, and bodily sensations as they arise so that we may helpfully address them before they lead us into fierce blocks or repetitions.

In this way, we become increasingly able to change as we wish with ever greater ease. Attending to our breath helps.

Following the Breath. In *shamatha-vipassana*, we place our attention on our breath. We notice the movement of air into and out of our body and the accompanying sensations of pressure and temperature. This is our mainstay for settling our mind. Unlike other techniques, such as focusing on a candle flame or another external object, we can attend to the breath wherever we are doing whatever we may be doing. We can observe our breath during an interview, in a conversation, making a presentation, saying our wedding vows, or elsewhere by gently drawing our attention away from our mental chatter and placing it on our breath. We observe our breathing carefully and respectfully. We may notice the temperature of the air moving into and out of our body. We may monitor the movement of our chest and abdomen as we inhale and as we exhale. Or we may observe the space between breaths. However we watch our breath we do not try to influence it in any way. We let it be. We simply observe (e.g, Kornfield, 1996). Zen Master Thich Nhat Hanh (2006) and Insight Meditation Teacher Sharon Salzberg (2011) also recommend silently saying "In" during the in-breath and "Out" during the out-breath to increase our concentration, which I myself have found extremely helpful in daily life. After three or four breaths, our breathing naturally begins to normalize, our mind is quieter, and our awareness resides primarily in the present. We see more clearly what actually is rather than imagining what is. We are better able to function as needed.

Learning to be with breathing this way helped me breathe rhythmically when I blocked. I realized, for example, I do not need to struggle to breathe, which only intensifies my fears about stuttering and, consequently, strengthens my tendency to stutter forcefully. What I do is to transfer my attention from the false belief that I need to fight to breathe to gently and non-judgmentally focusing on breathing *without trying to influence it in any way*. As I do, my breathing resumes its rhythmic, easy nature and so does my speech. It sounds simple. And it is. But it only became so after considerable meditation practice returning my attention to breathing when I noticed I was distracted by thoughts, emotions, and bodily sensations related or unrelated to stuttering. Building the skill of redirecting attention to the breath during meditation practice, where the emotional stakes are considerably lower than in everyday life, is essential to successfully doing so while stuttering (e.g., Silverman, 2006b).

Looking and Seeing: Vipassana

The difference between looking and seeing compares directly to the difference between the exactness of a realistic drawing made by an artist and one made of the same object by someone who is not. The artist has learned to see the subject of a drawing deeply enough to discern its individuality while the untrained individual has not. That is why an artist's drawing more nearly resembles the object drawn than an untrained person's whose drawing frequently seems to be a generic version of the subject. An artist, for instance, rendering a drawing of an ash tree may suggest the pattern and texture of the bark surrounding the trunk, the manner of attachment of the branches to the trunk and their relationship to one another, the shape and pattern of attachment of the leaves to the branches, the over-all shape and size of the tree, the tree's relationship to the surrounding environment, its age, and the season. Conversely, the untrained person who looks at the tree frequently seems to note it as a categorical object, i.e., A Tree. That leads to crudely portraying the individual tree as a caricature of itself with, perhaps, a rectangular shape depicting the trunk from which upward pointed lines of similar thickness suggesting its branches cradle an ovoid green shape representing leaves. Art teachers believe that learning to draw or paint realistically actually is a process of learning to see (e.g., Edwards, 1999).

Similarly, at least one meditation teacher refers to meditation as the inner art of learning to listen to what is happening inside and outside of ourselves (e.g., Kornfield, 1996). To effectively do so, meditation teacher and author Sylvia Boorstein (e.g., Boorstein, *et. al*, 2010) invites beginning students of mindfulness meditation to spend a moment before beginning each session choosing to meet each moment in meditation fully and to do so as though each was a dear friend. In this way, she explains, we are more likely to clearly see what is happening inside and outside of us and to do so without flinching, as we otherwise might, when we detect something unpleasant, which, like something pleasant, can occur at any time. This is the basis for non-judgmental observing.

Welcoming Thoughts, Emotions, and Bodily Sensations. Until we look deeply at ourselves and our stuttering, we will not know enough to respond skillfully to our stuttering. We will, most likely, react as we have done before with anger, fear, or disgust to the recognition that we are stuttering or to the impression we soon may be. If so, we resist. We refuse to talk. We stop speaking in mid-word or mid-sentence. We confidently or not apply techniques we have acquired to prepare for and manage our stuttering. Or we strain to push out sounds and words. Doing all or some of this, we may avoid or stop stuttering and feel relief for, perhaps, a nanosecond because we have survived what we consider an attack or a personal failure. But our momentary ease can readily become disheartening anguish as we recall we have experienced this relief before only to relive the struggle again and again. We can avert this emotional roller-coaster by calmly and closely observing our thoughts, emotions, and bodily sensations associated with our stuttering. That basic and critical decision can lead us to respond to our stuttering in a more skillful manner than to simply react. Therapy encourages a thoughtful response (e.g., Silverman, 2012), and mindfulness meditation practice shows us how. Like the artist who learns to look deeply to draw realistically, we can use mindfulness to look deeply to speak more effortlessly. Looking at ourselves and what we do as we stutter provides the fodder for speaking more as we wish, even as we stutter, if we first accept what we see.

During meditation, when we recognize, for example, we have been ruminating about how unfair it is that we have a stuttering problem, we can end that monologue immediately and return our attention to our breath. As we do, we forego self-recrimination because we recognize telling and retelling ourselves stories about what we have done or might do is what everyone does (e.g., Kabat-Zinn, 2005). In fact, rather than berate ourselves, we pat ourselves on the back. We recognize by noting we were distracted then immediately returning our attention to the present demonstrates we are choosing to be more mindful. Moreover, returning to the present in the midst of a reverie encouraging increasing anger, sadness, and, possibly, fear helps us learn to manage those strong emotions.

We can spend all or some of each session noting specific emotions and sensations in the body as they arise. We can gently dismiss them as we do thoughts to return our attention to the breath or we can attend quite closely to them, depending on what we believe is the best use of our attention at the time. Either way, we relate to emotions or sensations that arise with acceptance, even friendship. *"Oh, anger, there you are. I know you. I will take good care of you,"* is how Thich Nhat Hanh, Buddhist monk and meditation teacher, reportedly addresses anger and other emotions as he notices them arise (Hanh, 2003). *"Prickliness, Heat, Tingling, Itching"* are labels insight meditation teacher Jack Kornfield (1996) applies to bodily sensations he notes while meditating. Each affirms the appearance of emotions or sensations as natural, whatever form they may take. They do not react to them as hostile take-over attempts to be fought off or as failures of meditation to justify self-denigration. They simply note the emotion or sensation and decide how to best accommodate it, i.e., by immediate, gentle release or by study through deep seeing. And they encourage us to do the same.

We, with stuttering problems, can learn to apply what we learn in meditation practice while we wait to speak and even as we speak. We can quickly scan our mind to see whether we are caught up in stories we are telling ourselves about how awful it will be for us if we stutter. And, if we notice we are disturbing ourselves in this way, we can learn to do as meditation teacher Pema Chödrön (2004a) advises, which is to "drop the story line" immediately and return our attention to our breath. Doing so, we choose to be present and to be calm. Continuing our scan, we can note emotions we may be feeling and, rather than being ensnared, gently release them (e.g., Kornfield, 1996). Finally, but not necessarily in that order, we can note tightness or constriction in our chest, neck, mouth, or face and release the tension as we do when we notice uncomfortable bodily sensations anywhere in our body (e.g., Kornfield, 1996). The more we do this in our practice, the more easily we are able to speak with ease.

We learn we do not need to fight ourselves to change. Life is difficult enough, and fighting with ourselves only makes it more so. Resisting what we do not want to feel or do compounds our stuttering problem. What helps is first accepting, rather than resisting, what we are experiencing and doing no matter how disagreeable or upsetting that may be to us at the time (e.g., Kabat-Zinn, 2005; Kornfield, 1996). In fact, mindfulness meditation teachers, Tsultrim Allione (2008), Chöygam Trungpa (as cited in Gimlan, 2009), and Thich Nhat Hanh (2002) advise that desirable change follows when we warmly greet an emerging action we wish to discontinue by smiling inwardly to acknowledge its presence while silently re-affirming our choice to behave differently, then doing so. Likewise, Tsultrim Allione (2008) and Thich Nhat Hanh

(2002) apply a similar approach to managing difficult emotions as they arise. They silently address them stating they no longer fear them and will take good care of them, then they proceed to calm their minds. Through the process of staying described in the section which follows, they develop understanding and compassion for strong emotions. This is the basis for their willingness to work with rather than avoid them.

The poet Ranier Maria Rilke (Barrows & Macy,1997, p.119) advises that we all benefit from accepting what is, the agreeable and the disagreeable. He wrote:

". . . Let everything happen to you.
Beauty and terror.
Just keep going.
No feeling is final. . ."

His words remind us we embody change, or resistance to it. Our task like everyone else's is to learn to skillfully live with change. Knowing and accepting what we are experiencing is a start. At the very least, doing so leads us to challenge our beliefs about who we are and how we need to be (e.g., Silverman, 2010; 2005; Kubler-Ross, 1997).

Staying: Working with Shenpa

Shenpa, a Tibetan word, can be likened to an uncomfortable feeling we may have that signals things are not going as we wish. Being hooked by *shenpa* (e.g., Chödrön, 2003a), we experience the urge to flee by doing something to escape that uncomfortable feeling and what we believe it portends. A difficult word to define, *shenpa* triggers an "Oh-Oh" feeling that we are experiencing something unpleasant or soon will be. And that feeling pushes us into an accustomed *fight or flight* reaction that causes us to withdraw from the immediate, tighten, and shut down, a thumbnail description of our common reaction to feeling we may stutter. We may resist speaking, force out speech sounds we may be repeating or holding onto, substitute a word we believe will be easy for us to say for one we believe we will stutter, tune out, or all of that. By working with the *shenpa* of our stuttering to respond rather than react to what we feel, we face our fear with courage and curiosity rather than belligerence and become better able to skillfully work with it. We start by making friends with the *shenpa* of our stuttering.

Making Friends with The Unpleasant and The Pleasant. Our tendency as humans is to avoid or squelch emotions and sensations we are experiencing that we do not like and even those we do if we believe they will turn to pain. And, in the process, we create greater unhappiness for ourselves (Shantideva, *et al.,* 1977). Simply stated, what we do to be happy in the short term is often what makes us unhappy in the long run. For instance, we surf the web, graze through the refrigerator, drink, and so on to avoid unpleasant feelings, such as fear, anger, sadness, disappointment, resentment, irritability, boredom, and so on, that may arise when we feel alone or burdened. And these avoidance reactions can lead to addictions that can create even more unhappiness in the long-run. Those of us with stuttering problems know that, perhaps, the signature aspect of our problem is the way we relate to our fear and our dislike of stuttering in the moment. We avoid, we conceal, we struggle to squelch our stuttering, but we stutter nevertheless. Or we may refrain from saying what we want or need to say, another way of avoiding. Acting in these ways, we feel anger and shame, berate ourselves, and feel more anger and shame.

But we do not only resist uncomfortable feelings, we sometimes shut down pleasant ones as well. When we speak freely, saying what we want to say when we want to say it, we often, almost immediately, taint our enjoyment of speaking with the apprehension that sooner or later we will once again struggle. So, to circumvent experiencing that pain of leaving *fluency nirvana*, we say to ourselves, *"This won't last," "Just you wait; you'll be stuttering again," "This is a fluke,"* or something similar to dampen our enthusiasm, prepare ourselves to regress, and ward off the evil eye that brings disappointment if we experience joy and satisfaction. Fleeing *The Pleasant* sabotages our efforts to change just as surely as avoiding *The Unpleasant* because it, too, is an aversive reaction to fear.

When we anticipate stuttering or find ourselves blocking or repeating and when we are stutter-free expecting our stuttering to resume, we often behave similarly: We seek distance from our anxiety and physical discomfort. Professionals instruct us to not avoid our fears of stuttering (e.g., Guitar, 2005) because flight reactions grow our stuttering problem (e.g., Johnson, 1956). But we do not need to avoid our avoidance. Another response is available to us, one that we often would rather not consider, and that is staying with *The Unpleasant* and to *The Pleasant*. By staying with what makes us uneasy or even frightened, we learn to relate more skillfully to the root of our problem, fear, to move in a new direction. We learn our fear does not last; if it comes, it goes. And we learn we are not our fear and our fear is not us. By choosing to observe our fear with interest and curiosity, we recognize we are not what we are observing. We are so much more, and that realization can help us heal. We see and, perhaps, know for the first time that we do not have to succumb to an emotion, even a strong one. Knowing that we begin to believe we can speak and live more as we wish.

The thought of staying with unpleasant emotions and uncomfortable sensations may seem jarring at first since it is counterintuitive to our desire to avoid pain. We know that avoiding what we dislike provides temporary relief but it weakens us in the long run because we strengthen the belief we can not speak as we wish, and, by doing so, we fail to develop skills and resiliency that can accrue from facing social challenges. By fleeing stuttering, we diminish our opportunity to live as we wish. We may develop few friends because we shrink from opportunities to mingle. We may underachieve and earn less than we might when we opt for careers or jobs that place fewer demands on us to talk. And we may risk being dominated by partners we selected because they are talkative and minimize our need to talk.

And, paradoxically, the more we limit our opportunities to avoid guilt, shame, and self-loathing, the more we increase our vulnerability to being hurt. It is as if, by shrinking from what life offers, we risk becoming a target or magnet for what we fear (Chödrön, 2004a). The antidote is learning to do what we initially abhor and resist, staying. Standing toe-to-toe with the fears and the physical unpleasantness of stuttering from which we have fled much of our lives we apply our courage and curiosity to examine them (e.g., Kornfield, 2009; Allione, 2008). And we come to understand what the now-retired comic strip character Pogo meant when he looked at himself in the mirror and exclaimed with surprise and, perhaps, some relief, "*We have seen the enemy, and it is us!*" We recognize, irrespective of what is going on around us, it is, to a greater extent, our habitual thoughts and reactions that have and continue to beleaguer us. And, as we look closely, we see even they are not our enemies. They are not even us. They are part of the armor we don to navigate life as we believe it to be (e.g., Berne, 1996). Comprehending that, we realize we can release our speech sound fears, our word fears, our listener fears, our situation fears, and our expectation that we may never customarily speak as we wish. But how do we begin?

1. We do not seek *The Unpleasant* and *The Pleasant*. We simply welcome what arises as it arises. We do not have to look for; we only need to look. *The Unpleasant* and *The Pleasant* will present themselves in time.
2. We adopt a practice such as mindfulness meditation that provides a structure we can use to develop a helpful

attitude and useful tools. Sitting on a chair or cushion in *shamatha-vipassana*, after first calming our mind, we use our senses when a strong emotion we dislike arises. We seek to know it without interfering with its expression. We imagine its size, texture, temperature, color, its location in our body, and how it feels there. This knowing based on simple curiosity begins to dissolve our fear. We recognize we are watching and remaining unruffled. We are in its presence, in contact with it, yet safe. This awareness prepares us to learn how to respond skillfully with genuine authority. Likewise, when we experience tightness or breathlessness or fear, we bring our attention to the sensation or emotion and give it our similar attention (e.g., Kornfield, 1996). If or when this becomes too difficult for us, we return our attention to our breath.

3. We may partner with a professional. Learning to stay with challenging sensations and emotions is not a task to be undertaken lightly. Facing and learning to skillfully respond to well-established fears we may benefit from skilled and experienced direction and support.

Working with *shenpa* during meditation can help us learn to stay with *The Unpleasant* and *The Pleasant* and enhance tools we already possess to speak and live with greater ease.

Enjoying A Sense of Ease

When we live with ease, we glide rather than stumble along. We are on our game. But are we able to enjoy our new-found ease? That is the critical question. Mindfulness meditation teacher Thich Nhat Hanh (2006) said that if we are not able to enjoy being peaceful, then there is no reason to seek peace. Likewise, if we can not enjoy living with ease, there is no reason to seek it. We think we prefer ease to struggle but may be surprised to find that living in ease may be unsettling at first. We may find the relative quietness of living without fear of failure boring and the challenge of re-organizing our lives to accommodate new experience anxiety-arousing. If so, we may resume the struggle we know well. We may, for instance, invite worry, anxiety, anger, sadness, scheming, and other such pre-occupations back into our lives even though we know these states tie us in knots. But, like living in a run-down shack that may neither offer the amenities nor draw the admiration of a well-built, spacious residence, we have learned what to expect, and we feel more secure. Performing activities such as emptying containers placed throughout the house that fill with rainwater, shooing chickens out of crawl spaces, mending window screens, re-hanging doors to accommodate settling, and so on to create a semblance of order can bring a comfort of its own. Whereas, moving to a sound structure with minimal and, perhaps, unfamiliar maintenance requirements can prove challenging. To dull the anxiety occasioned by our new-found ease masquerading as emptiness, we may overeat, drink, engage in compulsive sexual activity, or escape the prickliness of our new, uncertain lifestyle in other harmful ways. Healthfully adjusting to a loss of the familiar that includes an increase in leisure time can be daunting until we recognize and acknowledge that such change brings the opportunity to live more as we wish and, then, do so.

Learning to enjoy a sense of ease speaking can be similarly challenging. Speaking without struggle, paradoxically, may generate considerable anxiety as in waiting for the proverbial other shoe to drop. We might recall, for instance, the times before when we spoke word-after-word, sentence-after-sentence with ease until once again we struggled to form and release sounds. These experiences led us to decide our new-found ease speaking earned through self-study, therapy, attendance at a workshop, or use of an electronic aid is only temporary, an interlude, until, once again, we know fear and struggle as an aspect of speaking. We may agonize that, while we can speak with greater ease, we can not do so at all times which leads us to live within a self-created conundrum where speaking with ease brings anxious anticipation, not satisfaction. Learning to live mindfully in the present helps alleviate the belief satisfaction breeds dissatisfaction. Even though we recognize nothing is permanent and we can expect to experience times when we stutter, we do not yet believe those times, too, are impermanent and that when we experience them, we can stutter without plunging irretrievably into everlasting struggle and shame. Through the tools we hone during mindfulness meditation practice, we can learn to skillfully manage such intrusive and false thoughts about our future that interfere with living and speaking with greater ease in the present.

Getting Comfortable. At the start of group meditation or when meditating with a tape, DVD, or online, the teacher may begin the experience by saying, "Get comfortable. Relax." Most of us find this difficult at first and notice that trying only seems to make it harder because we do not know in detail how we feel when we are relaxed. Eventually, after choosing to begin our meditation sessions with the intent to place our attention on welcoming our body sensations and labeling them with a single word, such as *relaxed, tense, tingly,* and so forth (e.g., Kornfield, 1996) rather than the instructions, *Get Comfortable* and *Relax*, we learn what it feels like to feel relaxed. After starting our sessions that way for a while, we then may be able to say to ourselves, "Relax," and feel relaxed because the word has become associated with the feelings of relaxation. We have forged a link between the word and the sensation so that the word can help trigger the sensations. That is when we can then use the word *Relax* as a *start button* to launch a course of helpful responses when we meditate and when we speak (e.g., Silverman, 2005

TWO MINDFULNESS MEDITATION PRACTICES FOR STUTTERING

L iving with ease, even in the midst of chaos, first became a reality for me as I learned to practice mindfulness in the forms presented in this chapter. After all, living with ease is one of the fruits of practicing mindfulness. Speaking with greater ease followed. So, as I learned to relate skillfully to my gripping fear of speaking up, especially through working with *shenpa*, I began asking for and giving advice under diverse circumstances, conversing, and arguing, all with a new-found spontaneity derived from the confidence my speech mechanism and I could hold up and would get the job done. And we did.

This change in my life and speech evolved despite my on-again off-again practice (e.g., Fischer, 2010). I first meditated in the early 70's for a few months to relieve the tremendous stress arising from building a career, maintaining a marriage, parenting, and running a household. Expecting the outer circumstances of my life to become more congenial but experiencing no immediate, discernable changes, I quit after convincing myself I could better spend the 20 minutes I meditated two times daily in other ways. I did not know then that the first changes I could expect would be inner not outer. In the '80's through the early '90's, even more stressed than I was earlier by dealing with a divorce from a colleague and by single-parenting, I resumed meditating relying on my sense of what meditation should be. Without the benefit of advice for growing a sturdy practice now available through accessible books, magazines, CD's, DVD's, websites, and podcasts and with no teacher, I relied on hope this drug-free, non-therapeutic practice of meditation would help me live a better life.

So, consistent with my lackadaisical approach to meeting my own needs, I sat to meditate every now and then. If I wanted a diverting interlude from work or family responsibilities or if I felt guilty for not having meditated for a while, I sat. Otherwise, I did not. This erratic approach resembled the path I followed years earlier when I began piano instruction as a young woman. When I practiced session after session without hearing or sensing improvement, I stopped cold for days or weeks at a time, resuming only when I felt a strong desire to do so. Surprisingly, when I did, my performance always exceeded what it had been at the time I quit. Somehow learning took place when I stopped trying to force it. And, so, it seemed, did ease with my meditation practice.

Nonetheless, if I now were to launch a practice, knowing what I know, I would practice daily, if only for 10 minutes at a time (e.g., Mipham, 2006; Salzberg, 2011), regardless of whether or not I witnessed improvement or whether or not I liked the experience because I have come to appreciate the power of discipline as an integral feature of creating desired change. But, if I practiced only now and then, I would not beat myself up since Zen Master Norman Fischer (2010) presents a convincing case for erratic practice being better than no practice at the outset. I would, however, examine closely why I was straying from daily practice.

With this overlay, I offer the following account of personal change not as a *paean* to myself nor as a roadmap for you but as an indicator of what the practice of mindfulness meditation can offer and what it demands for those of us who wish to speak with greater ease physically and emotionally. In a sense, this sharing of my experience practicing ancient mindfulness strategies, which originated in the East, thousands of years ago to help people like me live with greater happiness, offers nothing new. I made no modification of these practices which increasing numbers of people around the world follow (e.g., Boyce, 2011; Kabat-Zinn, 2005). I practiced them as I believe others do (e.g., Silverman, 2011; 2005; 2003). Then, I applied what I learned to how I stuttered and how I felt about stuttering. This, if anything, may be the novel element. I know of no one, who lived all of their life in the West, applying Eastern strategies to speak with greater ease. And, in this respect, I provide what may be a glimpse into what can be involved doing so for someone with a stuttering problem.

What is not novel is the recognition that we who have stuttering problems are more alike than different from those who do not. This awareness that we share a bond with others sneaks up upon us from time-to-time, as it does here, and merits deep reflection. All of us, whether we have stuttering problems or not and wherever we may live, seek to avoid what we consider unpleasant and, in so doing, unwittingly create more difficulty for ourselves. We overeat to avoid confronting people and circumstances that upset us and flirt with becoming obese. We drink to avoid facing fears and sorrows and risk becoming alcoholics. We become hoarders to the point of endangering ourselves because possessions in excess make us feel we matter. And we create stuttering problems for ourselves and, in the process, possibly forfeit a more spacious life for a cramped one because we believe avoiding stuttering may help us stop. Some refer to this universally human and troublesome tendency to escape what is unpleasant as a form of *shenpa* (e.g., Chödrön, 2003a). It was avoidance which was at the core of my stuttering problem and of many others' I have known (e.g., Silverman, 2005; Johnson, 1956). And it is this elemental and troublesome tendency being mindful can curb by helping us learn to non-judgmentally stay with what is.

To present a description of the mindfulness practices that helped me speak with greater ease, it is useful to first recognize and briefly reflect on the obvious and, maybe, the not so obvious:

1. *Applying mindfulness to stuttering depends on being mindful.*
2. *Being mindful derives from practicing mindfulness meditation.*

Meditation helps us develop the calm and penetrating aware-ness moment-by-moment that prepares us to become appropri-ately responsive, rather than customarily reactive, to our thoughts, emotions, sensations, and behavior and outside influences asso-ciated with our stuttering. While we may wish to speedily move toward our goal of speaking with greater ease by adopting the maxims of mindfulness, such as *relax* and *stay*, without adding the task of meditating to our already bulging schedules, we quickly find, as I did (Silverman, 2006b), we can not because: *Being mindful involves applying skills shamatha-vipassana meditation practice comprehensively develops.* And reaching this quality of mind and related quality of functioning can not be forced any more than tugging on the roots of a corn stalk can hasten the ripening of its ears. It is a process that grows with practice and by holding no expectation other than being increasingly aware of what is going on inside us and genuinely accepting of what is.

As we engage in the practice of mindfulness meditation, we do well to rely upon and, possibly, enhance the qualities we already possess of patience and of kindness. These help us develop the endurance we need since the process of becoming mindful is neither linear nor speedy. There are times we seem to be going backward and times we seem stationary as well, of course, as times we seem to be moving in the direction we wish. When we fail to notice desired change or, seemingly worse, when we notice ourselves relapse, we can become intensely frustrated. We may mercilessly berate ourselves for not practicing correctly or enough and, consequently, turn our practice into a combat zone. Or, reminding ourselves of our previous efforts to learn to speak with greater ease that failed to meet our expectations, we may convince ourselves to quit, concluding we should have known we can not be as we wish. To forestall such a hasty and, possibly, unfounded and harmful decision, we can draw upon our resource of patience and a practice of kindness to ourselves to bolster our resolve to keep doing what we believe will help and to do so for as long as it takes (e.g., Chödrön, 2003a).

KEY MINDFULNESS PRACTICES

Three forms comprise the core of my meditation practice. *Shamatha* meditation calms and steadies our mind. *Vipassana* meditation help us look deeply at what is going on inside out outside of ourselves. And *shenpa* work helps us remain moment-by-moment with what we perceive when we would ordinarily flee. Although I describe them as separate activities, they intermingle. But *shamatha* provides the foundation. Through it, we settle. That allows us to concentrate to look deeply into what is going on within and around us during *vipassana* meditation, which is the goal of that practice. And settling and looking deeply prepares us for *shenpa* work where we hone skills we already possess to stay with rather than avoid our stuttering and our fear of it. When staying becomes too challenging, I return to the practice of *shamatha* to settle once again.

Being calm, present, and accepting readies us to respond skillfully rather than habitually to our stuttering and our feelings about it. We come to recognize that without acceptance of what is as simply what is we can not change. We will not know in enough detail what we are doing or feeling to know what to change and how. *When we accept our stuttering and our feelings about our stuttering, we are not resigning ourselves to always stuttering and doing so in the same way.* We are setting the stage for responding in new meaningful and timely ways to be more as we wish. With acceptance, we bring gentle, skilled attention to our present thoughts, emotions, and behavior. In effect, we welcome them so that we know what we have to work with and how to do so. Without acceptance, we are likely to strengthen the accustomed thought and behavior patterns of denial, avoidance, and struggle we wish to change. As when we use *paradoxical intention* to work with what we fear (Frankl, 1959), accepting *the unpleasant* helps lessen, even eliminate, what we fear. I found, for instance, saying *Welcome!* silently as I felt myself stutter or when I believed I might, brought an almost instantaneous reduction of mental and body tightness and a reduction in the fierceness of my stuttering. I knew it was not the word itself that possessed the power to alter how I stuttered but, rather, the attitude and sincere belief embedded within it that stuttering could and would cause me no lasting harm (e.g., Allione, 2008).

These mindfulness meditation techniques foster calm and effective problem-solving (e.g., Kabat-Zinn, 2005). *Shamatha* calms our mind preparing us for *vipassana,* or clear seeing of what is going on inside us and outside us, such as our fear of rejection and of individuals' responses to us. *Shenpa* work develops the ability we have to stay with what we notice whether we like what we perceive or not so we can make the changes we wish to experience (e.g., Chödrön, 2005; 2003a). In the next section, we consider further the lessons and skills these practices offer someone with a stuttering problem. Those who wish to practice these mindfulness meditation forms may wish to consult the Resource section for materials and organizations that may help.

SHAMATHA-VIPASSANA: STOPPING AND LOOKING

One summer, many years ago, I walked around my neighborhood as speedily as I could almost every morning to unkink my skeletal muscles after writing for an hour or two. But every now and then something around me drew my attention, and I slowed down or stopped. A low-lying fieldstone fence, a vibrant blossom, the crunch of gravel underfoot, the acrid stink of freshly applied herbicide, or someone watering a flower garden jolted me into remembering life was bigger than I was living it (e.g., Silverman, 2010). Oh, I regularly scanned newspapers and magazines and looked at television to learn what was happening locally and beyond, but their focus on mayhem and tragedy began to convince me such was life, so I turned inward to escape the pervasive anger and sadness being exposed to those matters several times daily created for me. I made contributions to charities I thought might be offset the suffering I witnessed that helped turn my existential despair into a more hopeful outlook. And I spent moments looking ever more deeply into life around me to discover what I might do to enrich it and my experience of life.

Shamatha, the practice of stopping that helps tame the relentless self-talk of judgment, planning, worry, and regret common to us all, readies us for the clear-seeing we seek in *vipassana.* And, so, we practice them sequentially as if they were one extended practice. I often begin *shamatha* practice by attending to my breath after assuming a seated position in an area of my home reserved for practice (e.g., Kornfield, 1996). I observe where movement in my body is greatest when I am breathing in and when I am breathing out. I do not judge the location, range, or ease of movement. And I do not try to modify any movement. I simply observe with curiosity and interest how the breath moves into and out of my body and, sometimes, how it feels and seems. Doing so, I discover that this non-judgmental attention, seemingly of itself, encourages calm, steady breathing, and a calm mind helping me carefully observe with greater understanding what is going on inside and outside of me, the core of *vipassana* practice (e.g., Rosenberg, 2008).

During sitting practice, when I find my attention wandering from my breath, which, as for most practitioners, is often, I sometimes decide whether I have been thinking, feeling, or experiencing an emotion to heighten my awareness of when I am thinking or feeling or experiencing an emotion. Then I silently say *worrying* if that was what I had been doing, or *tingling* if that was what I had been feeling, or *sadness* if that was what I had been experiencing. If that seems too distracting, I just label the experience as thinking, or sensation, or emotion. At the same time, I gently disentangle myself from the story line I had been producing that provoked the experience. For instance, if I felt tightness in my lower back encircling my hips, I easily might have said to myself: *This position isn't right for me. No, that's not it. Yesterday I did more sit-ups than I usually do. I should have known better. I'll have to go easy for a few days. I need to pay more attention to my body when I exercise. If I don't I could really hurt myself. I can't afford to do that, not with all the work piling up . . .* I end such story-telling without self-recrimination since I have learned the nature of everyone's mind is to wander this way whether we are beginners or experienced meditators (e.g., Salzberg, 2011; Chödrön, 2004a). If I believe I might benefit from considering thoughts that arise, I decide to do so later. Then, I return my attention to the movement of my breath. *The over-riding goal in meditation is to experience what is present, not to think about it.*

As I was becoming increasingly well-acquainted with my breath during meditation, I became curious about how I breathed during daily life. So, occasionally, when I was standing in the check-out line at the supermarket, or sitting in my car waiting for the light to turn green, or waiting to see a physician, I attended to my breath. During those times, my breathing was deep, full, and continuous unlike when I stuttered or feared I might. Those were times, my breath was shallow, occasionally irregular, and sometimes, even, nonexistent, unlike the way I was accustomed to breathing as I meditated and when the specter of stuttering was not present. Experimenting, I observed that when I feared stuttering, I could place my attention gently on my breath with-out anxiety, judgment, or the intent to control it, as I did during *shamtha* practice, and be able to breathe more continuously and deeply and to struggle less if I stuttered.

Like others I return my attention to my breath over-and-over again when I meditate. When I first began to practice, I found this frustrating and, occasionally, boring. Later, after practicing for weeks and months, I sometimes found starting over this way demoralizing. When I began meditating, I thought nothing could be simpler than attending to the movement of my breath. Yet I quickly discovered I could only do so a few seconds at a time. I would place my attention on my breath and, almost immedi-ately it seemed, I would be planning or worrying or recalling or regretting, and I would have to start over. For months, session after session proceeded that way. I began to feel I had failed. I had not seemed to progress, and I became increasingly frus-trated. I wrestled with whether or not to continue doing what I believed was helpful but seemed beyond my ability. Unwilling to quit, I took frequent breaks, occasionally months at a time, then returned to practice because I believed I needed to be mindful to be happy. Eventually, I discovered that the abiding calm that was my goal could not be forced. It would emerge in its own way and on its own time-table.

I later learned through listening to CD's, especially those of Pema Chödrön, that every practitioner returns their attention to the breath again and again. That is an aspect of learning to calm and steady the mind. It is not a cause for regret. It is not a cause for becoming disheartened. And it is not a reason to quit. It simply is what everyone does. We practice the dictum: *I veer off-course. I gently return to course.* That is our central practice. And it is no less true when we work with our well-established struggle with stuttering. There we practice: *I am struggling. I gently release myself from struggling.* Each trip through this cycle taken mindfully brings us closer to more consistently speaking with greater ease and enjoyment.

Eventually, I realized how I relate to myself when I detect that I have let my mind veer off course is critical. If I silently scold myself for being "stupid," "hopeless," "undisciplined," or something similarly ugly, I sabotage my goal of change, since the subliminal message of such unconstructive epithets is, "You can't do it. Quit." But, when, instead, I use the recognition that by noticing I let my mind become distracted cue me to the fact I am learning to see how my mind works, I strengthen my resolve to attend and to treat myself kindly. So I choose to recognize mental drifting then resetting as acknowledgment of desired change rather than a sign of failure and as an opportunity to be kind to myself. Later, I generalized that reframing of the meaning of self-correction to the way I worked with my stuttering. I saw that resorting to hard struggle and knowing I could have stuttered with greater ease was recognition I knew I could change and I knew I how. And doing so kindly encouraged me to keep on helping me change from being a person with a stuttering problem to someone who simply stuttered now and then.

As I became accustomed to calming and steadying my mind to observe my body, thoughts, and emotions during practice, I found myself spontaneously applying those same, new-found skills during ordinary life. That surprised me. I did not know when I began meditating that the reason to practice was to apply the attitudes and skills learned through meditation to everyday life (e.g., Loori, 2008). I incorrectly assumed meditation was a quiet interlude that would incrementally infuse me with the calm needed to be stress-free, as if calm was an invisible protective cloak that would become increasingly likely to float down from the heavens and settle on my shoulders the more I meditated. But, occasionally, when I noticed myself steaming because I was stuck in traffic, impatiently waiting for a service call, or distressed in some other essentially, self-inflicted manner, I found myself remembering and applying what I was learning in meditation rather than stewing in the unpleasant feeling. I recalled I could be calm right there, right then. I could do something. Those thoughts, almost always, brought immediate relief and, sometimes, a relaxing smile. So, I disengaged my attention from the disturbing thoughts I had been entertaining, such as "I'm going to be late and miss the most important part of the meeting." "Why didn't I follow my instincts and take an alternative route?" "It was crazy to stop for coffee when I had so little time." and so on by silently and firmly telling my mind, "Clear." then focusing on my breath. That was when I knew my practice was helping me live more as I wished. Applying what I was learning to stuttering took more time.

Increasing Insight into Stuttering

The practice of withdrawing our attention from distracting thoughts and self-talk to be present frees us to deliberately look deeply into our present or past circumstances to discover what it is we need to do to be as we wish. By applying the clear sight cultivated through *shamatha,* we can engage in *vipassana* to work more skillfully with our stuttering. We may, for instance, deliberately revisit times we stuttered to see what was true for us about those experiences. We can observe calmly and without judgment what we did and what those around us did to draw insights we can use to speak with greater ease, then, at least temporarily, put those memories aside, where they are less likely to arise as intrusive events we re-experience repetitively to no useful effect.

Playwright Lillian Hellman (1973) made such pointed self-reflection the core structure of her memoir, *Pentimento.* She chose the Italian word *pentimento* as the title because, as she roughly defined the word, it means to look and to look again. She wanted to see what meaning experiences she had as a girl and as a young woman that shaped her life held for her as the mature woman she had become. As did Hellman, we, too, can benefit from reassessing our interpretation of memorable times. We can contemplate events associated with our stuttering when we were children to decide whether what we thought then was true about our problem we think is true now. And, like she, our success doing so depends on dispassionately observing, rather than reactively re-experiencing, those times.

Watching our recollections of those events unfold, as a curious but neutral observer during *vipassana*, we do not become blinded and ensnared by strong emotions that would arise if we were to relive those times. Rather, we view the circumstances in an expansive manner, to see all we can, rather than narrowly mining them for evidence to reaffirm our original conclusions. Viewing them dispassionately, we become free to notice how we postured ourselves, how we participated, and how we stuttered. And we observe as well those around us. We look to see how they presented themselves, how they interacted, and the timing and apparent circumstances of their comings and goings. We register particular elements of the scene, the season, time of day, lighting, sounds and sound level, dimension and accoutrements of the locale, temperature, and other apparent aspects that add to our understanding of the *gestalt* of the event. We turn our focus inward to recall our reasons for participating, our feelings doing so, the strategies we prepared, and whether or not we acted them out. Then, looking outward again, we gauge the possible effect our participation had on those around us and surmise the possible motivations they may have had that led them to behave as they did. What we are doing is analyzing the scene in a manner comparable to the way we might seek to understand a movie by considering the sets and the performances of the actors.

After dispassionately reviewing several remembrances of events when our stuttering was especially affecting for us, we recognize a certain core similarity in our thinking and behavior. We perceive, perhaps for the first time, the dynamic and pervasive influence of our fear, and we notice our instinctive response to our fear as resistance in the form of a fight or a flight response. That is common. As human beings, we instinctively want to vanquish what generates fear for us or escape from it. And we begin to see that so much of our stuttering problem stems from that very human response to fear. We take that in and understand perhaps more deeply than before what we need to do if we want to change. We conclude that to speak as we wish with greater ease requires us to skillfully manage our fear of stuttering and our correlated fear of speaking. And then we realize that staying with and accepting stuttering as it is in the present moment brings us closer to our goals of greater ease speaking, communicating, and living. That is where working with the *shenpa* of our stuttering comes in.

WORKING WITH *SHENPA:* STAYING WITH WHAT WE DISLIKE AND FEAR

Think about it. If you have a stuttering problem,

1. You do not want to stutter.
2. You do not want to put yourself where you may stutter.
3. You do not want to feel dominated by your stuttering. *And*
4. You want to beat it into the ground.

You want to be rid of stuttering. You can not imagine any other way of relating to it. That is why we rarely consider acceptance of our stuttering in theory or in practice as a first-order strategy. Yet, it is. And it is a key one. As I read Pema Chödrön's (2003a) article in *Shambhala Sun* magazine about working with *shenpa*, the Tibetan Buddhist term for how we get stuck in our lives, I recognized that my stuttering problem was a form of *shenpa*. It, too, was based in fear, strengthened by avoidance, and caused me to be stuck in my speech and in my life. The four mindfulness-based principles she presented as approaches to becoming unstuck resemble elements of techniques some have used to manage their stuttering (e.g., Fraser, 1989), so I was generally familiar with the principles underlying them. But the rationale and specificity of Chödrön's presentation gave me a new and fuller understanding of their usefulness and of stuttering problems in general. Collectively and singly, akin to practicing paradoxical intention (Frankl, 1959), Chödrön's *4 R's, Recognizing, Renouncing, Relaxing, and Resolving*, require a generous response to stuttering, which, for me, was challenging. But, I decided to apply them as I stuttered. And, *Voila!* My struggling continues to decline and my ease of communicating to increase (Silverman, 2005).

I was not able to apply the 4 R's to stuttering until I first did so with some skill and ease during sitting meditation, nor did I even consider the possibility. Learning to detect strong emotions while meditating, such as anger and fear, at earlier and earlier stages of their emergence by noticing accompanying changes in bodily sensations they precipitate, to see them as energy and *only* as energy, and then to witness their transmutation into a softer form of energy that gently dissipates when acknowledged and accepted is challenging for everyone (e.g., Chödrön, 2011b). But, after a while, my practice prepared and encouraged me to do the same in daily life with the anger and fear associated with stuttering beginning with the least challenging circumstances and working my way to the most challenging. And I slowly became able to do so, not all the time but enough to encourage me to continue the work. As with any other mediation-based learning, the timetable for skillfully applying these skills to stuttering to our satisfaction can not be predicted. But their steadfast practice during meditation prepares us for to apply them to our stuttering.

Practice is essential because, for me, and for most I have known, working with the body as a tool to skillfully manage strong emotions, such as fear and anger, has been a relatively unaccustomed practice. Cogitating is more familiar but more effective after we have experienced a troubling event when we can calmly examine our participation to learn what we might do differently from then on. But by working with *shenpa,* we discover that attending to the body is a sure path to change *in the moment.* While analysis helps us understand why we behave as we do and identify what we may need to do to be as we wish, skillfully utilizing sensations of the body as resources and guides to living skillfully in the present helps us *be* as we wish (e.g., Ray, 2008; Silverman, 2005). By working with the *shenpa* of our stuttering, we learn to utilize immediate experience for our immediate and long-term benefit of getting unstuck. This can be a marked departure for many of us from our propensity to think our way to speaking with greater ease. The *4-R's* of working with *shenpa* as I apply them to stuttering are:

Recognizing Resistance to Stuttering

The first step to getting unstuck is to notice and admit we *are* stuck. For me, the earliest conscious awareness of feeling stuck while speaking often has been the sensation of being grabbed by the front of the throat. It feels like what I imagine being choked by another might feel. I am startled, then frightened. I lose the sense of contact with those around me. I mentally interrupt the flow of words I intend to speak. My eyes widen. I hunker down preparing to struggle. My torso recoils. I stop breathing momentarily. Mentally, I demand to know what has brought about this ambush and why. No answer. I panic. I can not think my way out. I silently swear. I struggle to break free. I squeeze my eye and facial muscles and tense my thoracic and abdominal muscles to explode this word jam. I begin to sputter and spill out the crimped words and savor victory. My breathing becomes smoother and deepens. But, then, in a nanosecond, I crumple in shame. I resent the fact I stuttered and lost control of my body, again. The anger I feel feeds my personal discontent and can invite despair. I experience variations on this mind-body scenario based on my physical well-being and mental alertness in the moment. But all such scenarios arise from a forced manner of stuttering. And it is this forcing we can modify.

As do others with stuttering problems, I can become stuck even when I am not speaking but fearing I might need to speak. In fact, that was what led me to be selectively mute, *uber* stuck, for years. Urges to avoid speaking to avoid stuttering in certain environments, with certain people, and at certain times breed body sensations that send mind-body signals we can readily detect. For instance, I have learned through mindfulness meditation that almost as soon as I fear speaking, my throat constricts, the lower part of my stomach contracts, I squint, my heart rate increases, and the muscles at the base of my head tense. You may wish to take a few moments to observe how your body responds to the thought you may stutter. We each have our own way of responding to emotions with our bodies. So, we each benefit from becoming well-acquainted with our body's response to emotion. To experiment, find a quiet place to sit that is as free as possible from external distractions. Keep your spine erect, and place both feet firmly on the ground. Rest you hands palm down on your thighs. Then follow several breaths in and out of your body to quiet your mind. Settle. Image yourself called on in class or at a meeting to answer a question. Immediately introduce the thought, "I may stutter." Then scan your body. Look for any area that calls attention to itself. It may be tingling. It may feel warm, cool, tight, constricted, or otherwise that sets it apart. Then, without judgment, focus on that sensation as it is. Feel it fully. Get to know it. It is one of the early signs of fearing stuttering and, as such, a key tool for desired change. Repeat this investigation several times imaging yourself in different settings to discover whether and how your body responds to fear under different circumstances. For instance, you may wish to image yourself asking someone to dance or go on a date, purchasing an item, ordering in a restaurant, interviewing for a job, etc. Becoming acquainted and aware of these signals alerts us to change what we are doing on-the-spot by working with our body as an ally rather than struggle with it as a foe. And that helps us talk with greater ease.

Renouncing Struggling to Not Stutter, Not Stuttering Itself

Perhaps, more than once you were in a time or place where you believed you would be penalized for sneezing. Maybe you thought sneezing would lead you to be branded as a boor. Or, maybe, you were concerned about disturbing those around you, say at a wedding ceremony or at a movie theater. But even though you did not want to sneeze, your physiological need compelled you to. So, you conceded to the impulse with a determination to muffle the sound. You pressed your lips together tightly, held your breath as long as you could, and ducked your head to send the sound straight downward instead of all around you. Even, after all that, the sound was not to be denied and may, even, have been more explosive than it otherwise might. And we may have felt as badly as we feared, a bit of a failure for disturbing others and for not having squelched it. So we may feel bad for sneezing and bad for not containing it. We suffer twice! Contrast that experience with allowing a sneeze to exit without restraint The next time you feel the need to sneeze, allow yourself to sneeze, but attend to the feelings and sensations of needing to sneeze. Stay with the mental and physical tension, if any, and the closing down and withdrawing. Notice whatever emotions and sensations arise and morph while dismissing any discursive thoughts about them. Let the sneeze exit as it will. Maybe it will be loud. Maybe it will be a tiny squeak or a dull flutter-like sound. Then note how you feel afterward. You may feel less physical tension immediately and less guilt and shame than when you attempt to quell a sneeze and fail. Letting the sneeze be as it wanted to be, we only suffer once. But we suffer much less than half as much because we are not blaming ourselves for failing to do what we wanted to do. We may feel awkward and some regret for creating a small disturbance of no probable consequence. But we entertain no self-loathing. We recognize the sneeze as something people do. We know we need not feel guilty. Eliminating suffering for sneezing is one benefit that accrues from renouncing our struggle to not sneeze. Likewise, we can enjoy the similar relief from guilt and shame when we renounce our urge to resist a stutter.

Renouncing our reactive urge to resist stuttering, *not our stuttering itself,* is Step Two in working with the *shenpa* of our stuttering. After we recognize we might stutter and note we are reactively resisting stuttering we can act to eliminate the core of our stuttering problem, which has been defined as all we do to avoid stuttering (e.g., Williams, 1957; Johnson, 1956). In *renouncing* our resistance to stuttering, we do not repress or fight this unhelpful tendency. Instead, we welcome it, which, paradoxically, is the surer way to dissolve it (e.g., Boorstein *et al.*, 2010; Fehmi & Robbins, 2007; Hahn, 2003). For instance, when we detect bodily sensations that cue us that we fear we may stutter, we can silently renounce the urge to resist. We start by whole-heartedly welcoming it, which begins to dissolve the mental stress and muscular tension we have been building. Then we move forward literally and figuratively. We can choose to enter a situation or speak to a particular individual rather than avoid them. We can choose to look at rather than away from those around us. We can non-judgmentally watch our breathing rather than holding our breath. And we can continue talking rather than stopping as did a professor of mine in graduate school. When he stuttered on a word while delivering a lecture, which was quite often, he simply stopped saying the word and said the next one, or tried to. Note-taking was an almost futile activity. When we detect our urge to resist stuttering, we warmly acknowledge and welcome it as we would a dear friend and then we say what we want and need to say.

Responding skillfully to our emotions as we meditate prepares us. If we notice we are feeling an emotion as we meditate that we do not like, we do not deny it or push it away. We label it by silently tagging it "worry," "anger," "fear," "sadness," "resentment," "rage," "grief," "irritability," and so on (e.g., Kornfield, 1996). Then, we gently disengage our attention from the narrative we may be telling ourselves about this emotion we dislike and return our attention to the energy of the emotion itself, *separating raw experience from narrative*. We notice with a gentle curiosity how the emotion expresses itself in our body. Does it feel pervasive or localized?" Where do we sense it? Does it seem hot or cool? Does it feel tight or unbounded? We remain with these accompanying bodily sensation as long as they are present, gently and non-judgmentally observing. If the sensations become too uncomfortable, we can return our attention to our breath. We do not want to struggle with ourselves. We want to calmly abide. By learning to stay with what we fear or dislike, we are renouncing our customary urge to escape from or struggle with what we find unpleasant.

And conversely we do not struggle to cling to feelings we like, such as the satisfaction and, possibly, elation that we feel when we speak with more ease and assurance than is typical for us. For one thing, we can not. Good feelings like uncomfortable ones do not last. Feelings come and feelings go like the moments of our lives. And for another, trying to make a feeling we like last means we are resisting experiencing other feelings, which can include our fear and dislike of stuttering. And we know where that can lead. So, we remember everything is in flux, including sensations and emotions, even if we do not think so because we feel stuck in stiffening anger or grief that blaming ourselves and others for our stuttering problem can precipitate. And if and when we feel stuck, and most of us will from time-to-time, we can prove to ourselves we are not facing an impenetrable wall. We can practice *vipassana,* or insight meditation, to notice that anger and grief are not monolithic entities. They contain strands of sadness, hurt, fear, joy, and, perhaps, other emotions (e.g., Salzberg, 2011). Seeing that encourages us to believe we can work our way out in time.

Renouncing the urge to flee the possibility of stuttering, or stuttering itself, or the desire to cling to continue speaking free of our fear of stuttering when we do so, we proceed as we do as we meditate. When we detect bodily sensations associated with resisting fear of stuttering, we gently disentangle our mind from the feelings and any accompanying self-talk, such as *"Here we go again!" "Oh, no!" "Not this time!" "Damn it!"* and so forth. We do not run. We do not hide. We do not struggle. We mindfully say what we want and need to say. Relaxing helps.

Relaxing Into the Urge to Resist Stuttering and Into Stuttering Itself

When I was a student in the fifth grade, a classmate, smiling, challenged me to place my index fingers into the end of a short woven grass tube then pull them out. *How easy is that!* I thought. So, curious about why he asked me to do that but more interested in what might be an opportunity to have some fun during a boring class, I did what he said. Inserting my fingers into the tube was easy, as I had expected. But extracting them was another matter. As I began to pull them out, the tube began to lengthen, and to constrict around my fingers. Shocked by this unexpected and unwanted response, I panicked. I reacted by pulling harder to wrest them free. The tube, in response, lengthened even more and squeezed my fingers ever more tightly. They were trapped. I was certain of that. And I, too, felt trapped unable to imagine living with my index fingers stuck inside a grass tube. Seeing my distress, my classmate said kindly, "Push your fingers toward each other, then you can take them out." I did that. The tube widened. And I slowly and easily removed my fingers careful to do nothing to cause the tube to constrict again.

A while ago, while browsing through a puzzle store, I spotted a box of those tubes I had not seen since that memorable day in fifth grade. I bought more than few of them. Every now and then, when I was working with a client who had not yet made the connection between struggling to not stutter and having a stuttering problem, I handed him or her one of the tubes with the same instructions my classmate gave me. And, each person, after learning how to get unstuck, better understood that relaxing, by coming together rather than pulling away, is freeing because of what they, too, experienced.

Step Three in working with the *shenpa* of our stuttering , relaxing into what we do not like or fear to free ourselves of limiting thoughts and behavior, may seem mystical or *airy-fairy* until we recognize we have been developing this skill by practicing *shamatha-vipassana*. When we draw our attention back from enticing or disturbing thoughts, strong emotions, or palpable sensations to place it once again on our breath as we do during that mindfulness meditation form, we can relax into the distraction. We do not struggle to free our attention from it. We soften. We even may acknowledge the thought, emotion, or sensation with a sincere smile (e.g., Chödrön 2011b; Trungpa as cited in Gimian, 2010). The corners of our mouth, elevated slightly, suggesting a smile may frame the word "Welcome," silently uttered as though we were inviting a dear friend into our home (e.g., Boorstein *et al.*, 2010; Allione, 2008; Hanh, 2005). We fully accept this visitor as we enjoy our breathing.

Relaxing into our urge to resist stuttering, or stuttering itself, we exclusively focus on bodily sensations. We do not want to over-think what we are doing. We want to short-circuit our thinking to bypass our accustomed self-talk and the bodily tension it can create in order to soften. We concentrate on direct, immediate experience and our response to it. We focus on accepting the sensation of resistance. Then we sink into that feeling as though we were gently lowering ourselves into a hot bath. As we might yield to the warmth of the water, we let go. We feel tension melt. We feel at ease and move with less effort. This becomes more natural with practice.

Applying it on-the-spot takes some time. And we can not estimate how much. In fact, we do not seek to know because striving to meet a timeline can create unnecessary anxiety and related tension. We concentrate on conscientiously performing the strategy. Just as when we learned to ride a bicycle by practicing pedaling, steering, and braking without knowing when, or even if, we would be able to ride on our own and then suddenly did when our mind-body was able, we will know when we are ready to relax into our resistance to stutter, and we will. And also, like learning to ride a bicycle, once we learn, we will not forget. We have developed a muscle memory that remembers. In the meantime, we practice.

Resolving to Continue the Practice

Having experienced Steps One through Three, and noticing we have benefited from the practice, we resolve then and there to repeat the entire process as often as necessary to disrupt our habitual pattern of fighting stuttering. On paper, this step may appear the simplest of the four to enact, but it can become the most challenging. Most of us, once we commit to changing, want to consistently communicate as we wish *now*. When we do not, we flirt with reverting to our habitual avoidance patterns by entertaining such thoughts as, *"I can't do it right!" "Once a stutterer, always a stutterer!" "This is just another vacant promise!"* and so on. We find unsettling the uncertainty of whether and when the strategies we are practicing will enable us to consistently speak and live as we wish. To manage such nagging unease, we may try to convince ourselves that our old pattern of struggle is preferable to the effort, time, and suspense of an uncertain outcome of working with *shenpa*. Unless confronted directly, such fear-based thoughts can collapse our resolve to change. So, when we notice our thinking drifting in that direction, we stop. We cease such fear-based, defeatist thinking on-the-spot. We recommit to our choice to speak with greater ease by remaining rather than acting habitually on our urge to resist stuttering. We acknowledge that if we practice correctly and with diligence we are more likely to speak as we wish than not. We remind ourselves that, if we stop, the most likely outcome will be that we will behave as we always have with only with greater certainty that we have no viable alternative.

I learned that lesson many years ago, not in relation to stuttering, but by learning to restructure my life to lose extra body weight. Highly motivated for an ingloriously compelling reason, I scrupulously followed the food selection, caloric consumption, and physical exercise guidelines and the firm injunction to weigh myself only once each week outlined in the pamphlet my physician gave me. For the first several weeks, I enjoyed eating less and exercising more because I reveled in the downward sloping line forming on my weight-loss graph. But when I lost no weight for two successive weeks, I was shocked, then furious! Fairly ignorant about the process of losing weight, I did not know such plateaus represented the body's need to stabilize. I chose to believe this stoppage meant I would never lose all the weight I wished. That conclusion generated bitter thoughts: I felt angry that I had raised my hopes only to dash them once again. I felt sad believing I was doomed to lug around a body unattractive to most. And I felt frightened concluding I lacked control of my body. I railed at the unfairness of not getting what I thought I had earned and stormed around the house shouting, "I'm going to quit." But my husband at the time convinced me to stay with the program. He patiently explained without condescension that if I continued eating and exercising as I now did, I would continue to lose weight. Not doing so was contrary to the laws of nature. I knew what he said was indisputable, so I continued, although somewhat skeptically because I irrationally believed that somehow I might be an exception. I was ready to quit at the first sign I could not lose more weight. But, of course, I continued to lose more weight except during two or so additional week-long plateau periods in the nine months ahead, and I maintained a stable weight for more than 10 years until I decided to adopt a vegetarian diet. Again, with only scant information to guide me, I fearfully bulked up on eggs and dairy products to ensure I was receiving enough protein and gained eight pounds That spurred me to learn what constituted a healthy lacto-ovo-vegetarian diet. I developed one for myself, followed it, and returned to the weight I enjoyed.

I began applying the 4 R's to my stuttering without much forethought. It seems that watching my mind and taking corrective action to stay with rather than escape what I did not want to engage with during meditation became an increasingly strong response that transferred to ordinary life, stronger, eventually, than many of my well-habituated reactions to flee literally or metaphorically. I instinctively began choosing to stay when I detected myself beginning to avoid stuttering. When I did, I felt the parts of my body that had been resisting or struggling soften. And I felt my mood lighten, as when a heavy concern fades. My stuttering lost its fierceness. I repeated less and, when I did, I repeated sounds and words more smoothly. I activated my vocal cords with greater ease. Blocking ceased almost as it began. Mentally, I remained more in touch with the people and circumstances around me. I felt connected with rather than apart from others and from life. I felt hopeful that finally I could actually fit in and be happy.

If I were to begin doing *shenpa* work now specifically to learn to respond skillfully in everyday life to what I consider unpleasant as well as to what I judge to be pleasant, I, as a speech-language pathologist, might follow a structured plan to apply what I was learning in mediation to stuttering. I might, for example, begin the process by reciting lists of common knowledge, such as the days of the week, the planets in our solar system, or the names of the months or I might count from one to 100 or count from 100 to one for a greater challenge to my concentration and cognitive processing, while observing myself in a mirror and introspectively. I would attend gently to body sensations alert to feelings of tension/ease, tight/spacious, warmth/coolness, prickliness/smoothness, and so on as I spoke, when I stuttered and when I did not. By observing myself in real-time rather than while watching video tapes, I would learn to attend to body sensations as I spoke, noting which tended to precede, coincide, and follow stuttering, which did not, and which coincided with not stuttering. Attending closely to sensation is what we need to do to strengthen our ability to recognize opportunities to make timely adjustments to speak with greater ease as we speak and to simultaneously weaken entrenched, disruptive mental and emotional reactions to speaking and stuttering that might surface. But I would not deliberately change how I was speaking until I had completed the next two categories of tasks:

1. When I was comfortable with rote activities, which require limited linguistic planning, demand no social communication skill deployment, and stimulate little to no emotion, I would continue the practice of attending to body sensations while verbalizing more personal matters. I might, for example, describe the room I was in, the route I had taken to work, the strategy I used to mow the lawn, or any such circumstance devoid of strong emotion.

   Again, I would speak as I looked at my image in a mirror, preferably a full-length one. My goal would be as before, to amplify my attention to body sensations as I spoke, using visual feedback to help, if necessary. When I could, I would up the *ante* by inducing myself to experience strong emotion, particularly apprehension. I might imagine myself speaking up for myself in a circumstance where I could expect censure, or, at least, dismissal. For instance, I might imagine myself asking my supervisor for a raise, telling my partner what more I needed from our relationship, refusing an invitation to join a neighborhood group devoted to gossip, and so on. All the while, I would monitor what I was saying and how I was expressing the message through facial expression, body posture, hand and arm gestures, and vocal tone and, especially, the sensations in my body.

2. When I felt able, I would repeat these final tasks by adding two critical features: I would instruct myself to renounce resistance to stuttering and, when I stuttered, to relax into the stuttering using imagery or by smiling sincerely as a statement of welcome to the stuttering.

Contributing significantly to whatever benefit I might realize from these exercises is how I relate to myself as I performed them. Relating with the kindness and respect I deserve in the tradition of *maitri,* or unconditional friendship toward myself (Salzberg, 2011; Chödrön, 2009) considered in some detail in the following chapter, encourages us to persevere to be more as we wish. On the other hand, relating to myself with annoyance and contempt for not yet being as we wish delays the possibility.

But, I might not follow such a plan or any plan. Doing so would provide too strong an enticement for me, a seasoned competitor, to concentrate more on outcome than on process, and, given, the uncertain timing and nature of the outcome of working with *shenpa,* lure me to quit before I reaped benefits from the practice. Another reason is that I approach life intuitively (Myers, 1995; Jung, 1976). I prefer to be open to process rather than locked into following a pre-arranged plan. So, knowing what I know, I probably would proceed in the manner I did. Not only is that strategy more in keeping with my personality, it is, I believe, more in keeping with the practice of mindfulness and working with *shenpa,* in particular.

As we know from watching a sunrise or sunset, change in nature is constant but not easily noticeable moment-by-moment. This is just as true for personal change. For instance, when we peer at our face in the mirror, we rarely see daily differences in our skin texture, hairline, and muscle tone unless they are quite marked or we are especially alert. Instead, we see our face as our face, unchanged and, essentially, timeless. But, we know better. We know we do not look as we did when we were 13 or 23 or 33 because we have photos to remind ourselves. We changed from year to year. We simply did not notice the process underway day by day. Similarly, when practicing *shamatha-vipassana* and work with the *shenpa* of our stuttering, we may not recognize changes preparing us to speak more consistently with greater ease until they reach critical mass status. And we can not predict when that may be. So, we resolve to be steadfast. If we are uncertain about the adequacy of our practice, we may want to consult with a teacher or with resource materials.

When we do noticeably start to change, some of us may feel uneasy. We can not foresee how our lives will be We become fearful. We wonder: Will our work and personal relationships change? How will that affect us? Will we live somewhere else? How will that affect us? These concerns remind us that when we change how we speak, we change how we communicate and that can alter how we live. When we see that change is not only possible but happening, some of us may ask ourselves: Am I ready to change (e.g., Myss, 1999)? If our answer is "No" or "I don't know," we may behave as a woman I met when I was an undergraduate student clinician. She stuttered severely by silently repeating the first sound of almost every word she spoke while baring her front teeth looking like a snarling dog about to bite. She had learned many techniques to stutter with greater ease and could demonstrate them all when asked, but she was unwilling to use them in her daily life. When I asked why, she shrugged her shoulders as though surprised to be asked and replied, "They don't feel natural." At the time, in the early 1960's, these techniques constituted the core of stuttering therapy offered by most speech pathologists. So, her reason for continuing to attend therapy seemed not to change but to satisfy some other needs, perhaps, for affiliation, which the director of the therapy program apparently supported. We will not know. What we can surmise is that, from a speech mechanics standpoint, she did not need to stutter as she did. Perhaps, she eventually did not as she learned, as we all do, that we only feel comfortable with new behaviors after we have practiced them for some time so that they feel like old behaviors.

How long it can take to learn to speak with greater ease is uncertain. What is certain is that our consistency practicing correctly with a clearly stated and genuine intent moves the process along. And applying the four supplemental mindfulness practices presented in the next chapter can strengthen our resolve and further direct and maintain our focus.

6

FOUR ADDITIONAL MINDFULNESS PRACTICES TO PROMOTE CHANGE

Having had a stuttering problem and having worked with many who have, I have come to believe that misunderstanding and underestimating who we are comprise our greatest impediments to speaking and living with greater ease (e.g., Silverman, 2010; Chödrön, 2009). When we reflect on how we relate to ourselves, we often see we behave as though we were the stuttering we detest rather than the capable people we are. This self-vilification deepens and widens our stuttering problem by encouraging a false sense of separateness and, occasionally, a sense of hopelessness that can accompany feeling alone in the world. Conversely, relating to ourselves as friend can help transform our life into an up-beat, grounded adventure that, while it may have highs and lows, can lead to living a more expansive life. Incorporating the ancient Buddhist practice of *maitri,* unconditional, positive self-regard, into our mindfulness practice along with three other established meditation practices, namely *lojong,* the reciting of *gatha's,* and *tonglen* can help us live mindfully to experience greater ease. Altogether they infuse the practices of *shamatha-vipassana* and working with *shenpa* with tools to help maintain and strengthen our practice in the face of the many pushes and pulls of daily life.

While I discuss these four as though they were individual activities, they function as elements of a whole practice that helps us live with greater clarity, purpose, and self-regard. It is as though *shamatha-vipassana* and working with *shenpa* were the hub of a wheel whose spokes are *maitri, tonglen, lojong,* and the recitation of *gatha's.* The combined practice helps us see more clearly into and develop skills to relate more skillfully to what is.

MAITRI: CULTIVATING UNCONDITIONAL, POSITIVE SELF-REGARD

Maitri is a more concentrated version of *metta,* or friendship (e.g., Salzberg, 1996). When we practice *metta,* we learn to relate to all beings, including ourselves, with compassion and kindness (e.g, H.H. the Dalai Lama, 2006). When we practice *maitri*, we cultivate unconditional, positive self-regard or friendship toward ourselves, which we in the West often seem to overlook as critical to living as we wish (e.g., Salzberg, 2011; Chödrön, 2004a). Until we consider ourselves deserving and capable, we are unlikely to believe we can live with greater ease and to make the necessary effort to do so.

Far from encouraging selfishness, *maitri* encourages our consideration of others. Learning to be more compassionate toward ourselves, even when we stutter, we learn to be more understanding and compassionate of others, even those who knowingly or unknowingly cause us pain. In this way, practicing *maitri* helps us create conditions and circumstances that allow us to experience life in a more congenial way. Doing so, we speak and live with greater ease.

Relating to ourselves with love may not only be our due but our duty. The Buddha taught, *"If you search the entire world, you will find no one more worthy of well-wishing than you."* His message that we are no better or no worse than any other being and that all of us deserve to be related to with kindness at all times resounds through the Judeo-Christian scriptures as the directive "Love your neighbor as yourself" (Leviticus, 19:18; Mark 12:30-31), one of the two principal commandments concerning everyday conduct. This five-word directive instructs us to love ourselves and to do so first and foremost and unconditionally. We are to love ourselves for no other reason than we are. It does not matter what we do or do not do or how often or infrequently or how well or how poorly we do it. We are told to love ourselves. From this perspective, we differentiate our behavior from our nature. If we believe we are behaving in ways that may be harmful, we change to do what is helpful instead believing we are capable and deserving of living with greater ease. We do not love ourselves more when we have done what we think is well done or less if we believe we have not done well. We love ourselves unconditionally and steadfastly because we recognize doing so not only helps us live with greater ease but others as well. Consider the following Hasidic tale I have modified slightly:

Some time ago, on the eve of the Jewish New Year when acts of charity have special merit, a rabbi living in an Eastern European village solicited donations for the poor. When he visited the home of the local miser, the man as usual, declined to give, stating that the poor should make greater efforts to support themselves. He shouted he would not support laziness. Deftly changing the subject, the rabbi asked why he, who had the means to live comfortably, lived in such a mean way, residing in a hovel that was dark and dank. Without hesitation, the man replied, "This is enough for me."

Through thoughtful conversation, the rabbi encouraged the man to enjoy his wealth instead of hoarding it. And he did. He built himself a sturdy home. He ate fine foods and drank good wine. He purchased a silk brocade suit for himself and satin dresses for his wife and daughters. He enjoyed his wealth. The following New Year the rabbi visited the man at his new home to again request a donation to improve circumstances for the poor. This time the resident gave readily and generously. And that became his custom from then on.

"How was it" the rabbi's wife asked, "that he changed so radically?"

"When he lived as a pauper," the rabbi explained, "he did not realize how difficult the life of the poor was. Once he moved into a sound home, ate and drank well, and dressed himself and his wife and daughters fashionably, he knew."

How we relate to ourselves can make our lives heavens or hells.

Maitri sometimes is translated as *lovingkindness* (Chödrön, 2009; Salzberg, 2005). Practicing *maitri* we commit to creating happier and more peaceful lives for ourselves and for all others. Starting with ourselves, we offer ourselves unconditional, positive regard. This differs from indulgence. Indulgence is escapism not kindness. When we practice *maitri*, we introduce ourselves to constructive beliefs and provide our bodies with adequate nutrition, hydration, rest, exercise, and kind attention so they feel and function better. And when we appreciate the way they serve us, acknowledging, for example, that our eyes help us see so many wonderful things, our feet help us move from one place to the next, our arms carry things, our teeth help us eat the food we need and enjoy, and so on, we seem to function in a more graceful and efficient manner. But if we berate ourselves when we make a typo, hit a wrong key playing the piano, or stutter, we do not necessary type more accurately, play music more satisfactorily, or speak more easily. In fact, the disapproval we show ourselves may lead to additional typing errors, extra false notes, and more stuttering.

When we relate to ourselves with kindness, we function more smoothly, we make desired corrections in our beliefs and behavior more assuredly, and we are happier. If we can not readily convince ourselves we are worthy of such positive self-regard, as many of us in the West whether we have a stuttering problem or not often can not, we need to look more deeply. When we make the effort, we usually can find one reason we deserve our kindness and well-wishing. It may be that we would not hurt another to make ourselves feel better. Or, that we once wrapped a one dollar bill around a one hundred dollar one to slip it without ado into a Salvation Army kettle at Christmas-time. Or we removed snow from the front walk of a neighbor who was ill even though we were cold and wet from removing snow from our own property. Or we stayed up late one Christmas Eve when we were tired to help a friend wrap presents to give the next day. When we identify at least one such action we have performed or intention we have held, we recognize that as a reflection of a quality, such as humility, generosity, or charity, within us. And, if we can not find one reason for wishing ourselves well, we may recognize that the fact we are searching to do so is reason enough (Salzberg, 2005; 1996).

Searching for aspects of ourselves we find praiseworthy can be an unfamiliar and uncomfortable activity for those of us living in the West where society encourages us to believe we are never quite right. We remain on the lookout for aspects of ourselves that interfere with embodying society's image-ideal to feel acceptable and accepted rather than to detect and embrace our strengths. Such continuous, critical self-scrutiny can create self-loathing, whether we have a stuttering problem or not (Silverman, 2009), that can impede or even stymie our efforts to change to be as we wish.

Practicing *maitri* reduces self-loathing by helping us balance and expand our awareness of who we are. When we practice *maitri,* we recognize we possess desirable qualities and attributes, not just unacceptable ones that surface when we look at ourselves, as we customarily do, through the lens of "someone who has a stuttering problem," or some other limited and limiting self-concept (e.g., Silverman, 2010). Practicing *maitri,* we seek to acknowledge and embrace all of ourselves (e.g., Silverman, 2010; Myss, 2008; von Franz, 1964), that which we admire and that which we detest. Doing so, we are choosing not to live in denial by pretending all is well with us *or* that nothing is good about us. Practicing *maitri,* we experiment with our attention to see all we are, the praiseworthy and the regrettable (e.g., Salzberg, 2011), to embrace it all to heal (e.g., Whitney, 1985). By practicing well-wishing for ourselves, we acknowledge we are worthy of greater happiness not because of our thoughts or behavior *per se* but simply because we are.

During *shamatha-vipassana* meditation, while working with the *shenpa* of our stuttering, and wherever and whenever helpful, we practice *maitri* by silently offering wishes for our well-being. Starting with ourself we recall how fundamentally alike we all are. Not only we, but all beings, wish to be happy and live in peace. After we become comfortable well-wishing for our personal happiness and ease, we do so for all manner of beings: Those we like. Those we do not really know or know well. And, eventually, those we find difficult. Mindfulness meditation teachers Sylvia Boorstein (2010; 2008) and Sharon Salzberg (2011; 1996) suggest we formally practice *maitri* by expressing the following wishes, or similar ones, in a heart-felt, focused manner:

1. *May I live free from danger.*
   We affirm our wish to live free from external dangers, such as muggings, bombings, fire, robbery, drive-by shootings, floods, and so on, and from internal dangers, such as self-deprecation.
2. *May I experience mental happiness.*
   We affirm our wish for our lives to be satisfying and meaningful through challenging and well-paid work, caring relationships with partners, family, friends, and associates, resiliency, and freedom from nagging existential concerns.
3. *May I experience physical well-being.*
   We affirm our wish for health, strength, flexibility, and endurance.
4. *May I live with ease.*
   We affirm our wish that in matters of family life, work, friendships, and casual relationships we be free from struggle.

As we include others, we may specifically name those for whom we are offering these wishes or identify a group of beings for whom we are offering them, such as *all those who feel misunderstood* or *all who feel rejected, etc.* Tibetan Buddhists believe thinking of others in this way facilitates our own healing (e.g., Mipham, 2007).

The fruits of this practice, as do the fruits of *shamatha-vipassana* and working with *shenpa*, present as they will, often slowly, sometimes imperceptibly restoring an inherent grace to our lives. The first sign I detected I was becoming more compassionate toward myself was approximately one week into the practice of *maitri*. I found myself silently cautioning myself in a kind, yet firm, voice, "Don't be mean to me." as I ripped into myself for dropping my toothbrush onto the bathroom floor. Surprised by the intercessory words I never before addressed to myself, I ended my hurtful tirade instantly. I smiled. I knew right then I was changing, and I knew in my gut not just in my head that continuing to behave cruelly to myself was foolish.

Ever since, I find myself silently vocalizing such encouraging phrases such as "It'll be all right." "What needs to get done will get done." and "It's OK." when I do not perform as I wish or when circumstances confound the realization of my desires. I readily accept this self-generated feedback then relax, instead of pushing and forcing to have my way. I do not necessarily cede my goal. I calm my mind so I can thoughtfully decide whether, when, and how to try again. This approach to dealing with obstacles helps soften my muscles, including those of my tongue, jaw, chest, and abdomen; deepen my breath in quiet and while I speak; and release me from the thrall of impatient and perfectionist demands I may impose upon myself. And, unlike times past when I could spend hours disappointed with myself after failing to meet my expectations becoming increasingly despairing of my ability to live as I wished, I spend little time regretting failures. Instead, using the skills I am developing through the practice of *vipassana*, I look deeply into challenging situations to discover the best way to keep on keeping on.

Relating With Kindness to Ourselves and to Our Stuttering

There is romantic love, parental love, love of work, love of friends, and love of country. Loving prompted by neediness can provide the highest emotional highs and the lowest emotional lows, while selfless love can lead to serenity. We can love one another, animal companions, an ideal, the earth, and all of creation. But without kindness and respect we do not love; we hurt instead.

Learning to love myself, I am learning to love my stuttering. While stuttering is not an "other," we often think of stuttering that way. In fact, we commonly refer to our stuttering as "It" (e.g., Williams, 1957). When we do, we objectify our stuttering: It is not us. It is something foreign. And many of us, from childhood on, believe our stuttering is something that can assail us. So we often relate to our stuttering as we would an adversary from which we flee. We act as though we are playing a game of tag running from the one we call "It" to feel safe. But our stuttering is not an "It" chasing us or any other kind of "it." *Our stuttering is what we do.* So, if we run from our stuttering, we run from ourselves (e.g., Silverman, 2010). Running we park our attention in the past or propel our attention into the future and risk behaving mindlessly in the present. Running from ourselves we impair our ability to communicate convincingly in a timely manner. We do not win when we play the game of "It" with our stuttering

Conceptualizing our stuttering as an "It," which we often begin doing as children when our life experience is limited and our thinking apparatus immature, can jump-start a lengthy process of feeling stuck in our lives. By relating to our stuttering as an adversary that can attack and over-power or destroy us at any time, we may live within a small space to feel safe. We may believe limiting the possibility we may stutter by speaking as little as possible to as few people as possible under as few circumstances as possible will minimize rejection and the pain that can bring. But, eventually, we discover this strategy diminishes our enjoyment and satisfaction rather than increasing our happiness. Then we may allow our anger and resentfulness to become bitterness.

Like those in Plato's allegory living inside a cave chained in such a way that all they could see were the shadows on the wall in front of them of who or what passed by, we, too, experience only a semblance of life when we restrict our mobility. But, unlike Plato's cave dwellers unaware of what they were missing, we realize we experience less of what is available to us when we withdraw. And we can feel sad and angry and become depressed. That is likely to be what we experience when we mistakenly believe our stuttering is an entity and one more powerful than we until we realize we put the chains on ourself and we can take then off.

Some ways we communicate the false belief our stuttering is an "It" is by telling ourselves and, perhaps, others:

It (stuttering) just happens.

I wish *it* (stuttering) would just go away.

Why did *it* (stuttering) have to happen to me?

By repeatedly entertaining these beliefs, we wire them into our unconscious where they can create a fomenting sense of helplessness and hopelessness that can breed undercurrents of sadness, anger, hurt, and rage fanned by the angst arising from an often held companion belief that by giving us a stuttering problem life has treated us unfairly. These reactions, when unchallenged, can prevent and sabotage efforts we may make to speak with greater ease. We may, for instance, eschew speech therapy, rationalizing that since it did not heal us as children, it probably will not help us as adults. We may enroll in speech therapy only to stonewall it so we can demonstrate to speech pathologists, with whom we may be angry because we believe they failed to help us when we were frightened and trusting children, that they lack the knowledge and skill to help people with stuttering problems. We may uncritically align with professionals, products, and services that offer to transform our stuttered speech into non-stuttered speech and risk becoming prey for those seeking to use us to satisfy their personal needs for recognition and financial gain. Or we may seek the company of those who support our sense of feeling like an outcast from society because we stutter increasing our already sadness and anger, since that self-concept, even though painful to hold, may be more comfortable than embracing the unknown self we may encounter when we change. What we will *not* do, if we believe our stuttering is an "It" is learn to speak with greater ease with increasing consistency or abandon the mantle of "Outsider."

Assuming the role of neutral observer to closely examine my involvement with my stuttering as well as that of my clients' convinced me stuttering was not an "It," as speech pathologist Dean Williams (1957) argued so long ago. I saw for myself what he, also someone with a stuttering problem, knew, namely that we create our own stuttering problems. I tensed the muscles of my face, tongue, and torso to not stutter when I was afraid I might, which increased the possibility I would. I struggled to push out sounds and words as I stuttered, then stuttered all the more fiercely. And I lived in fearfulness that I might stutter, which lead to fashioning anger and hurt as prevailing emotions. That is what we all tend to do and what we all tend to experience when we believe our stuttering is a faceless enemy we call "It," an outside force stronger than we that we believe is intent on attacking our personal sovereignty.

After looking carefully at what we do when we stutter, we can appreciate what the now-retired comic strip character Pogo realized when, anticipating a war, he stared at his reflection in a full-length mirror and saw that, "I have seen the enemy, and it is us." *Our stuttering is not an "it;" it is what we think and do.*

We recognize through our practice of *shamatha-vipassana* and, perhaps, from our knowledge of theories for constructive personal decision-making, such as, general semantics (e.g., Johnson, 1980; Korzybski, 1955), transactional analysis (e.g., Berne, 1996; Harris, 2004), or cognitive-behavioral therapy (e.g., Segal, *et al.*, 2002; Ellis and Harper, 1975), or from honest self-reflection (e.g, von Franz, 1964) our thinking and our use of language interrelate to structure our lives. It has been suggested that we do not describe the world we see. We see the world we describe. So, to live as we wish, we learn to examine our use of language to verify that it faithfully reflects the view of this world and our place in it that we know to be true.

So, in the manner comparable to honoring a unifying peace pact we might sign with an adversary to end a prolonged, hostile, winless engagement, we can choose to love our stuttering by according this falsely identified former foe kindness and respect. We accept our stuttering whenever and however we stutter without a tad of complaint to ourself or to anyone else that we stuttered or that we stuttered in a way we did not like no matter how inconvenient or embarrassing we believe the stutter to have been. We refuse to tie the heavy anchor of complaint around our ankles to bob up and down and risk drowning in waves of anger, fear, or hurt when and because we stutter. We choose, instead, to sail on. We relax into our stuttering. Allowing our stuttering to be as it will we stutter less and with greater ease.

We also accept the anger, fear, and hurt associated with our stuttering as we do our stuttering itself. Accepting rather than shooing these emotions away, ignoring them, or stuffing them into our unconscious because we do not like relating to them, which is common whether we have a stuttering problem or not, helps them dissipate (e.g., Allione, 2007). Unwelcomed, they burrow into whatever part of the body-mind they find a congenial host. From there, camouflaged, they can relentlessly instigate challenges the way a bratty child lurking behind the railing of a second story porch may wait to spit on hapless walkers below. By acknowledging their presence, then looking deeply into them, we learn to work with them as we might learn to help our child when he or she comes to us shouting and hurling accusations, sobbing, or looking glum.

When our child arrives distressed, the most important thing we can do is to offer our kind attention. We acknowledge the child's pain. We draw our child close. We encourage our child to be. And when our child ready, he or she may tell us what we can do to help or quietly leave. But our child already has felt some relief by being recognized and accepted (e.g., Allione, 2008; Hahn, 2005). But, if we ignore him or dismiss our child because we are uncomfortable relating to anger, fear, or hurt, his and ours, our child may return again and again exaggerating the pain until we notice and help. If, after all that, we do not and our child becomes convinced we will not, our child may behave outrageously to provoke us to offer our attention even though our child knows our attention may take the form of anger, which our child may prefer to no attention at all. Similarly, our anger, fear, and hurt, when we fail to acknowledge them, may morph into especially unpleasant versions of themselves, such as dark moods, fatigue, sarcasm, increased and increasingly forced stuttering, and, even, illness to garner our attention when we do not heed the message they bring about our beliefs.

Loving ourselves and accepting our stuttering, we live and speak with greater ease. We no longer live at the ready to evade or ward off every stutter. We soften. We replace walls we may have placed between ourselves and others to spare us rejection with openness. We see and accept ourselves and others more fully. We feel safer and stronger.

LOJONG: FOCUSING USING SLOGANS

When The Going Gets Tough, The Tough Get Going. Keep Your Eye On The Prize. No Excuses. These slogans and others like them can jump-start our intent to change and keep us going as we run into challenges learning to be as we wish. That is why we use them. Almost as we hear, see, or recall them, they lift us out of any zombie-dom we may have slipped into the way a tap on the shoulder can awaken us from a daydream. We might apply them then and there or not until later, but, at the moment we notice them, they galvanize our attention and revitalize us.

They inspire us to take constructive action by inviting us to live more purposefully. Through a few easily remembered words energizing to repeat that may take the form of plays on words or stirring lines from poems, songs, or scripture, they help free our consciousness from numbing distractions that reduce our energy and dampen our enthusiasm to rouse us to action. The seemingly universal dictum, "Do unto others as you would have them do unto you" may be the granddaddy of all slogans. For that reason, champions of reform, politicians running for office or re-election, manufacturers, service providers, and religions rely on it or its derivatives, such as "Do not ask what your country can do for you; ask what you can do for your country," to act in accord with their higher aims.

Tibetan Buddhists have long utilized *lojong* practice to help awaken or re-awaken themselves from the slumber of forgetfulness to take helpful action. Brought to Tibet from India *via* Sumatra by a monk called Atisha to cultivate self-love, or *maitri*, as the primary step toward relating to others with genuine compassion (e.g., Chödrön, 2011a), *lojong* practice involves heeding 59 slogans first codified in written form during the 12th century by the Tibetan Buddhist monk Geshe Chekawa. Pithy, they function as stirring reminders to apply the teachings to everyday life and as directions for doing so, the gist of mind training (e.g., Chödrön, 2011a; 2004b; Hahn, 2011; Loori, 2008).

We, too, who intend to speak with increasing ease, can benefit from using slogans that remind us how we intend to communicate in everyday life and how we can do so. These engaging reminders smooth our transition from hiding and struggle to more open communication (e.g., Siegel, 2010a: Begley, 2007). And I have discovered 5 of the 59 (e.g., Chödrön, 2007) especially pertinent to working with stuttering problems. The five remind us to honestly and courageously address my beliefs about speaking, stuttering, and the process of change. They are:

1. *Change Your Attitude, But Remain Natural.*
2. *Abandon Any Hope of Fruition.*
3. *Liberate Yourself By Examining and Analyzing.*
4. *Don't Wallow In Self-Pity.*
5. *Don't Expect Applause.*

The meaning of most seems self-evident, such as *Liberate yourself by examining and analyzing*, but others, such as *Change your attitude, but remain natural* and *Abandon any hope of fruition,* may seem enigmatic. Yet each helps us learn to communicate with increasing ease.

Change Your Attitude, But Remain Natural

Thought precedes behavior, as those who adopt creeds know. When we avow our core religious beliefs during congregational worship or recite our societal ones in unison with members of a secular group, we do so as a reminder to act in accord with our beliefs. But, although we readily can recite religious creeds and group credo's, we often have difficulty remembering our deeply personal beliefs about ourselves, others, and the world because, by the time we are adults, they reside in our subconscious. Yet with determination we can excavate them as we work our way out of a tendency to relate in ways that antagonize those we care about or as we change the way we relate to things, such as food, drink, and the internet. As we examine beliefs that lead us to behave in ways we now wish to change, we find that although we adopted them to relieve our pain they caused us hurt. We recognize, for instance, that though we decided to avoid stuttering to be accepted doing so has caused us to feel isolated instead. Weeding out the unhelpful belief we need to stop stuttering to be accepted by replacing it with the recognition that we can stutter and still fit in since we all are members of the one human tribe helps as much as anything else we can do to speak and live with greater ease.

Replacing unhelpful beliefs with helpful ones, we come to relax, which is the meaning Chödrön (2007) ascribes to "remain natural." Buddhists consider relaxation our natural state, to which we can return though meditation and mindfulness. *Shamatha-vipassana* develops the skills we can use to relax wherever we are. For instance, mindfully attending to our inhalations and exhalations to calm and stabilize our mind readies us to more clearly experience our emotions as the energy they are without being pushed and pulled around by them. Through our practice of *shenpa,* we learn to sink into that emotional energy as if it was a tub of pleasantly warm water where we experience the energy then feel it dissolve leaving us calm and relaxed, which we can do whether alone or in the company of others. Similarly, when we notice ourselves beginning to resist stuttering, we can sink into the bodily sensations associated with that struggle. We scan our body to find the energy we label struggle, or resistance. Then we slide into it as if it were a cozy bed on a cool evening. We imagine ourselves pulling up the covers and relaxing into the sensation by refusing to tell ourselves any stories about the sensation. We release words and embrace sensation. We relax. And we can do this on-the-spot having practiced this technique during *shamatha-vipassana* meditation

Because our new-found self-knowledge can liberate us from excessive self-consciousness and other unhelpful behaviors to avoid being hurt, we can choose to be grateful for detecting our misperceptions about what we need to do to live and communicate with greater ease. For instance, Pema Chödrön (2011a), when teaching *lojong*, suggests we be grateful to everyone, including ourselves, who have hurt us in one way or another because each hurt provides an opportunity to analyze and examine our beliefs and behaviors bringing a springboard to change.

Abandon Any Hope of Fruition

Living as we do in a culture that impels us to routinely ask, "What is in it for me?" we are likely commit to a plan to change only if we can visualize a desired payoff for ourselves. Signing-on without expectation of personal gain, such as communicating more as we wish, seems strangely counter-intuitive and, probably, unappealing. Even though we may have other motives, such as quelling our mother's voice in our head that we do something to stop stuttering or basking in the empathic interest of winsome, empathetic student therapists at the local university speech clinic, we still are likely to involve ourselves in a program only to satisfy our desires.

The apparent paradox of foregoing personal expectations while striving for personal change resolves when we recognize the essential message is a reminder to live mindfully by focusing on what we think and do rather than on what we want.

It is reasonable to begin a program of change to satisfy a desire. In fact, why else would anyone begin? But, once we begin, focusing on our ultimate goal rather than participating in the process to get us there can be a grave distraction that can fuel impatience. And that, in turn, may impel us to quit if we believe we are not getting all we need as quickly as we wish. When we wonder how long it will take for us to speak with greater ease in restaurants, at meetings, on the phone, asking for dates, shopping, and so on, or whether we ever will, we squander the time available to us to fashion the outlook and skills we need to communicate as we wish. Worse yet, we can create enough doubt about our ability to change to sabotage our undertaking. Our goals inspire and direct us. But what we *do* changes us.

For some, when we or others note signs of we are changing, we can mistakenly assume we are able to stop stuttering and be as we wish everywhere and always. But that belief, too, can derail our change process. It can be a corollary of the belief we must not stutter. Whether we focus on avoiding and suppressing stuttering directly or indirectly we distract ourselves from our overriding goal of communicating well with ourselves and others, and we risk serious disappointment. Extending the time we communicate with greater ease is a gradual and non-linear process. Attending to the process of becoming mindful of what we think and what we do moment-by-moment helps us become more as we wish. We commit to engaging in the process of mindful speaking rather than striving for a specific outcome. We recognize by attending to process we can reach our goal of communicating with greater ease the way we are likely to successfully complete a lengthy trek by mindfully placing one foot before the other rather than wondering about what we may encounter along the way.

Liberate Yourself By Examining And Analyzing

When we decide to carefully examine how we approach speaking and how we approach stuttering and how we speak, we are taking responsibility for learning to consistently speak with greater ease. And we are announcing to ourselves and to those tuned in to us that we are in charge of our change process. We are no longer depending on others to tell us what to do. We did when we were children and teens because we thought parents, teachers, therapists, and other adults knew what was best for us and, perhaps, because we though we had no other choice but to do what they told us to do. But, as adults, we no longer need to cede our power to others to shape us as they will. Becoming well-informed and taking responsibility for how we speak and stutter is our task. We may consult with those who may provide helpful information. But we decide whether, when, and how to use it.

Assuming responsibility, we release ourselves from living in anger and resentment that believing another has to control us can incite. And, in the context of assuming responsibility, we refuse to blame anything or anyone, including the universe and ourselves, when no one or nothing seems to intercede on our behalf when we encounter difficulties that overwhelm us. Blame wastes time and energy available to be as we wish and risks stalling our change process. We choose to become more pragmatic. We search for a path to lead us to our goal. We may consult with those who have knowledge and skills we need but have not yet acquired, but we do not relinquish the position we rightfully assume as the one charting our life.

We know by thoughtfully examining and analyzing what we do, we can identify what beliefs and behaviors help us communicate as we wish and which do not to do more of what helps and less of what does not. But, paradoxically, for a brief time, we may opt to do more of what we do not want to do to consistently speak as we wish. This is the premise behind *paradoxical intention*, a self-help technique popularized by psychiatrist and logotherapist, Viktor Frankl (1959). Frankl discovered that giving ourselves permission to carry out a feared activity in an exaggerated manner helps eradicate our fear and reshape our behavior to our liking. He related the experience he had with a physician who became fearful of performing surgery because he sweated profusely while operating. Frankl advised him to give himself permission not only to sweat while operating but to sweat enough to fill buckets during the next surgery he performed. The surgeon accepted the suggestions but, not surprisingly, could not sweat as Dr. Frankl demanded. That ended his fear of excessive sweating while operating. Similarly, speech therapists sometimes suggest to individuals with stuttering problems that they stutter deliberately in situations, at times, and in ways they do not want to stutter. This pretending, referred to as voluntary stuttering (e.g, Guitar, 2005), helps reduce their fear of stuttering and their felt need to avoid stuttering.

Don't Wallow In Self-Pity

For most of us, things go wrong from time-to-time. We fail to get what we want or feel we deserve or we get what we do not want and feel we do not deserve. This can come in the form of challenging individuals or circumstances that appear in our lives creating obstacles and triggering memories of similar situations in which we felt hapless and, even, defeated, providing additional opportunities to feel inadequate, angry, or resentful in the present. And, given the cyclic nature of stuttering, we find ourselves from time-to-time stuttering more intensely or more often and panicking (e.g., Guitar, 2005). We revert to accustomed strategies to avoid stuttering. We may leave a room, clam up at a meeting, or even inaccurately report the results of our own research findings during a thesis defense, and so on.

This can happen even though we are learning new beliefs and behaviors because they do not yet possess the strength and resiliency of the fear-based ones we wish to replace (e.g., Siegel, 2010a). We may feel angry at ourselves. We may think we could have thought and acted better. We may feel scared. We may believe we can not change, that we are doomed! And we may feel sorry for ourselves that we have to work hard to speak like others who speak without apparent effort, and, even then, we still stutter. We can wallow in self-pity. But that is not going to help us feel better or be as we wish. *Wallow* is the operative word. We acknowledge we are feeling sorry for ourselves. We even welcome the feeling as we do all feelings (e.g., Boorstein, 2008). We examine the thoughts and beliefs that dispose us to feel that way, eliminate or modify those we have learned are unhelpful, and remind ourselves of those that better serve our intent to speak with greater ease. Then we go on. We resume doing what we believe helps us speak and live as we wish, acknowledging we will not always act or think as we wish especially during challenging times when older beliefs and behaviors are stronger than the ones we are learning. And we acknowledge that we can restart the process at any time without the need to feel guilt or shame (e.g., Salzberg, 2011). We keep on keeping on. We have neither the reason nor the time to feel sorry for ourselves.

Don't Expect Applause

Change to satisfy yourself, and you will be happy. Change to satisfy others, and you will not. Others, allies and adversaries alike, may recognize, ignore, or fail to notice what we are doing or have done to feel better. They may commend us. They even may ridicule us. It makes no difference. When we do what we know we need and want to do, we will find satisfaction regardless of how others react or respond. The only opinion that matters is our own. It is our life after all. Learning to live it for ourselves we become strong.

I rarely accepted an adult as a client who wanted to enter therapy primarily to satisfy someone else, such as a parent, part-ner, or an employer, unless I believed the client was willing, but frightened, to change. To fear change is common. That can be worked with, but entering therapy primarily to satisfy some-one else's wish or demand adds a phantom third player to the mix that can sidetrack or derail the enterprise. Using therapy to act out power struggles and other unresolved issues rather than attending to learning to speak with greater ease can eas-ily sabotage therapy. Clients driven to address someone else's desires for them may stonewall therapy to gain revenge while simultaneously strengthening their personal belief that speaking with greater ease is unattainable for them. And by doing this they do little to mitigate relationship problems at home or at work that they could by directly addressing them, possibly with advice and direction from a mediator or counselor.

In a lighter mode, we might imagine the sound of one hand clapping. This is a well-known *koan*, or Zen verbal puzzle that has no logical solution. Imagining such a sound can help remind us to change for ourselves and *only* for ourselves and that our personal opinion of ourselves is the one that matters. We might visualize a forearm and hand moving from side-to-side in front of our body as if clapping. If we do, we might smile, even chuckle, because we see.

Reflecting further on this slogan, we realize that unless we are acting in a play or skit, performing a monologue, doing a stand-up comic routine, debating, or speaking publically in some other way, we are not performing. When we speak at home, work, in a church or synagogue, in a store or restaurant, on the street, or elsewhere, we are talking to people who seek information, direction, comfort, encouragement, or, at least temporarily, human companionship. As a story teller explained, it is the telling of a story as much or even more than the content that captures and moves an audience or not. That is just as true when we speak with others. When we interact with those around us putting their need to be informed or comforted before our own to speak without stuttering, we can be engaging. If not, we may be off-putting and discomforting. So, if we notice we are first and foremost seeking to be known as someone who can produce mechanically flawless speech, we immediately refocus. We charge ourselves to connect instead. Later, we can look deeply into our motivation primarily to perform rather than to connect at that time to better understand why we were seeking acceptance from others rather than establishing fellowship with them. Then we practice *maitri* with the intent of increasing self-acceptance, which, we may be coming to realize, is the only form of acceptance that contributes to lasting happiness

As slogans do, after we contemplate them even briefly, these five may pop into our consciousness at just the right time to help us remember what we need to do for the long haul. Some people begin each day with the intent to observe a particular slogan (e.g., Chödrön, 2007). The next day they observe another, the day after that a third and so on until they complete their list of slogans. Then they start over again. If we do not want more daily "to-do's" in our life, we can let these slogans enter our consciousness as they will. Their surprise visits help us commit to continuing our practice to speak and communicate with increasing ease.

GATHAS: FOCUSING THROUGH VERSE

Like using efficiency experts' suggestions, applying *gatha's*, or short verses, while meditating and throughout the day can reduce unhelpful expenditure of energy. As we recall or recite them, *gatha's* guide us in ways to live with increasing mindfulness. But, unlike slogans, which, once we have adopted them, can enter our awareness serendipitously without apparent effort on our part and, in the process, momentarily stop our minds from free-wheeling, *gatha* use requires us to first deliberately stop thinking. To appropriately apply them, we first rein in our attention to place it squarely on an object of attention, such as a thought. We acknowledge the thought for what it is, namely a thought, and, as we do in *shamatha*, we release it and added-on story lines. We stop worrying about what might happen. We stop regretting what we did or did not do. We stop resenting what was said or done to us. We stop all ruminating. We settle. Then we recite a *gatha* silently or aloud that pertains to what we intend to do, such as making a phone call (e.g., Hahn, 2006a). Reflecting on the words, as we might in *vipassana*, we become more clear-sighted envisioning then approaching and carrying-out the task. Using *gatha's*, we better appreciate how our thoughts and actions can contribute to the arc of our life and the lives of others.

Gatha's remind us there is no task too small to bring us happiness and satisfaction when performed mindfully. There are *gatha's* for sweeping, watering the garden, turning on the computer, driving the car, using the telephone, eating, moving, resting, in fact, for most activities of daily life (e.g., Hahn, 2009; 2006a), as well as for activities requiring sustained effort to realize a long-term goal, such as working for unilateral disarmament (e.g., Hahn, 2009) and helping children meditate (e.g., Hahn, 2010a). One *gatha*, the *gatha* for conscious breathing, which facilitates the mindfulness meditation practices of *shamatha-vipassana* and working with *shenpa*, can be used to speak with greater ease (e.g., Hanh, 2009). Other *gatha's*, such as those for smiling at our anger and letting go of attachments, also use conscious breathing as framework and also can help us speak and live with greater ease and satisfaction.

You may wonder whether applying the *gatha* for conscious breathing differs from practicing *pranayama*. *Pranayama,* sometimes called yogic breathing, uses the breath to control the life force, i.e., *prana* (e.g., Rosen, 2010). The *gatha* for conscious breathing facilitates normalization of breathing. For instance, using the *gatha*, we first stop. Then we silently recall it:

Breathing in, I know I am breathing in.

Breathing out, I know I am breathing out.

- - - (Hahn, 2009, p. 4)

We recognize we are breathing. Noticing we are breathing in when we are breathing in and knowing we are breathing out when we are breathing out stabilizes and calms our mind while allowing our breath to naturalize in the manner of diaphragmatic movement seen in a healthy infant lying on its back. We notice our in-breath, and we notice our out-breath. That is where we place our attention. We watch, perhaps, ever more carefully with each successive cycle, noting the temperature of our breath, the depth of our breathing, the accompanying movement in our chest and abdomen, etc. But we *only* watch. We make no effort to control or change the way we breathe in nor the way we breathe out, nor do we wish to. And we do not hold our breath as we might during certain *pranayama* exercises. Using the *gatha*, we relinquish voluntary control of the process. We allow our breathing to be as it is. We just watch with interest.

Practicing *shamatha-vipassana* to carefully observe thoughts, feelings, and emotions as they express themselves through my body, I noticed I, as do others, hold my breath when I am fearful and, sometimes, when I am quite angry. And I also observed that by returning my attention to breathing, often with the help of the *gatha*, I resume breathing, a little jerkily at first, but, as I continue watching, I see my breathing become smooth again. Not surprisingly, after practicing *shamatha-vipassana* for some time and becoming more interested and skilled in observing my thoughts, feelings, and emotions during daily life, I noticed I hold my breath when I am afraid I might stutter and, often, as I do. Once I made that observation, I began to apply what I was learning during meditation when I noticed I was holding my breath.

On the spot, just as during meditation, we can return our attention to our breath and do so without editorializing. We concentrate on watching our breath, not controlling it. We observe and accept what we notice. Within several seconds, as we gently observe our breath going into our body and out of our body, we feel calmer. The mental chatter disappears. We are more aware of what is going on inside and outside of ourselves, and we feel more confident about doing what we need to do. Gradually, we become more adept at focusing in daily life as we do during meditation. Reciting the *gatha* for conscious breathing helps us to settle and to speak with greater ease. We even may smile.

TONGLEN: CONSIDERING OUR CONNECTION WITH OTHERS

There is an old Buddhist story which starkly depicts how similar we all are. Here is my version of it:

A woman became inconsolable after the death of her son. She neither ate nor slept and clutched the boy's body against her chest. After some time, her concerned family and friends encouraged her to meet with a wise man visiting a nearby village hoping he might be able to help her care for herself and bury her son. The woman sensing their love for her and wanting help agreed to go.

"Master," she said, reverently sitting before the calm, attentive man. "Please help my son. I implore you. Make him live again."

The man replied softly, "Return to your village. Visit each home to find one person who has not known death and bring that person to me."

The woman's heart warmed. "This I can do," she thought.

Until dusk that day and from dawn to dusk the next, she walked from hut to hut along the dusty roads. But after she visited the last dwelling, she still had not found one person to bring to the wise man.

She felt disappointed, then sad. But then she knew: Death comes to everyone. She walked into the field and buried her son.

The wise man was The Buddha who taught nothing is permanent. We all experience loss of people, things, and hopes, and we suffer. Yet we can learn how to skillfully free ourselves from our suffering. The woman in the story represents us. Like she, we, too, suffer when we believe we are different and alone. Those of us with stuttering problems know this well. We can feel separate and apart as we observe people around us chatting, joking, and enjoying carefree camaraderie because unlike most, including family members, co-workers, neighbors, friends, and salespeople who we presume say what they want when they want, we can struggle to say even our own names. Along with the shame and embarrassment we feel being unable to say something as straight-forward as that when we wish, we can become increasingly frustrated because we do not know why.

I knew a research scientist, someone with a vast knowledge of stuttering and a considerable knowledge of speech therapy, who somewhat facetiously proposed "The Poltergeist Theory of Stuttering" to try to ease his frustration at being unable to understand why he was one of the relatively few people who have stuttering problems. He speculated that poltergeists, mischievous spirits, made him stutter by zapping his tongue with electromagnetic rays to amuse themselves watching his struggle to speak. Maybe poltergeists did torment him, and maybe they did not. But, when we stutter, we, too, can feel attacked and different, especially when we are children and, often, the only one we know who has a stuttering problem. We may believe there are two kinds of people in the world, people with stuttering problems and everyone else. And, since we recognize those of us with stuttering problems constitute a very small minority, we may come to think of ourselves as aliens, the way 10-year-old Jason, the lead character of *Jason's Secret* (Silverman, 2001) only somewhat facetiously refers to himself. And we often carry this belief with us through our teen years and into adulthood wondering all the while whether we ever will be "normal," which, through our pervasive doubt, deepens our belief we will not. Eventually, though, most of us learn what we do is not who we are and that doing what it takes to be so-called "normal" may or may not be what we want in the long run (e.g., Silverman, 2010).

From a certain and increasingly well-known perspective, we are all alike in our essence no matter what we do or do not do or what we believe or do not believe. That is the message the Dalai Lama widely shares (e.g., 2006). He reminds us we all are the same because we all want to be happy and not to suffer. Even when we hurt ourselves by eating to excess or starving ourselves or through shoplifting, compulsively gambling, hoarding, refusing to speak to avoid stuttering, and so on, we can recall we began doing so to be happy. We thought engaging in these acts to evade feelings, sensations, and emotions we considered unpleasant or possibilities we feared we would not suffer.

And that is what we discover about ourselves and our stuttering problem. After looking deeply and courageously into how we relate to our stuttering, by using skills we develop practicing *shamatha-vipassana*, we see that all that we do to avoid stuttering comprises the essence of our problem (e.g., Johnson, 1956). Evading people and situations and sounds and words, pushing through a stutter or suppressing one, holding our breath or exhaling with force all generate misery, not happiness in the short- and long-run. Recognizing we are running from rather than facing what we fear we can feel shame and guilt. We blame ourselves for being weak. We think of ourselves as cowardly. Our self-deprecation grows when we act to avoid stuttering. And lacking self-esteem, we fail to believe we deserve better. We may not seek help or fail to fully engage in the process to change ourselves if we do. Eventually, recognizing we lack skills to communicate with ease and enjoyment because we have not developed them by conversing with a variety of people in a variety of circumstances or acquired other speaking skills, such as interviewing and giving presentations, to advance ourselves at work because we avoided opportunities to develop them to avoid being witnessed stuttering, we contribute to our suffering by increasing our feelings of loneliness, bitterness, and, possibly, unworthiness.

Ultimately, though, our desire for happiness by avoiding suffering unites us with everyone else. Everyone, whether they have a stuttering problem or not, knows suffering, knows rejection, knows disappointment, and knows the anxiety uncertainty can bring. Yet, we rarely acknowledge this similarity. Instead, we fixate on how we differ from everyone else because we have a stuttering problem. We overlook the reality that those without stuttering problems also know the pain of feeling different. Failing to see our common bond exacerbates, even creates, our problem. Seeing our common bond helps us heal.

Perceiving ourselves as different can lead us to consider ourselves outsiders vulnerable to rejection. This perception can cause us to live fearfully and harbor resentment. And, if we view our outsider status as permanent, we suffer greatly. To protect ourselves from such hurt, we frequently withdraw from those who seem unaware, indifferent, or callous to our pain and even from those who seem especially self-confident, if their assurance encourages us to feel inept. When we do interact with family, co-workers, acquaintances, and strangers, we may don a poker-face to look cool rather than anxious or expectant or we may act jovial and agreeable to conceal our anger and hurt. We fail to recognize that false and transparent posturing ratchets-up our vulnerability to those looking for someone to taunt or to con by communicating our strong desire for acceptance and our fear of rejection.

We may believe that we will suffer less if we minimize our contacts with others. We may seek comfort from associating primarily with those we consider more like us, for instance, people who also have stuttering problems. But eventually we realize shrinking our lives does not relieve our suffering; it increases it. By isolating ourselves, we can become prey for those who exploit the unhappiness and insecurity of others. And we can feel hopeless to the extreme. We may discard, for example, our lives of pain and, possibly, take the lives of others as acts of revenge or spite when we choose to believe no one cares or understands how much we hurt and never will. While that may or may not be true, everyone knows the sorrow life can bring, even those who appear unaware or callous of the pain of others.

When we look deeply, we can see those around us also are suffering. Just as the woman in the story, we may come to recognize there is no one we may meet or know who is not acquainted with the pain of loss. It may be through separation from a beloved partner, child, friend, caring neighbor, or other dear one, such as an animal companion, or through the loss of home, job, aspirations, reputation, or health. Feeling alone magnifies this pain and can encourage as us to transform it into deep suffering. Yet, as the woman in the story, we, too, can release ourselves from such suffering by recognizing our solidarity with those near and far and relating to all, especially to ourselves, with compassion and love.

We Are Not the Only One

Tonglen, the meditation portion of the *lojong* mind training program, helps us dissolve our sense of isolation and the suffering it supports by revealing through the deep awareness that w*e are not the only one* (Chödrön, 2003b). We are not the only one who hurts by feeling misunderstood or unappreciated. And we are not the only one who hurts by experiencing the pain of rejection. Others we know and others we do not also hurt for the same reasons. As members of the one human tribe, we share the totem of suffering. We all suffer, but we can release ourselves from our suffering. This bad news/good news circumstance forms our ineffable human bond. Recognizing suffering as common and inescapable, we cease feeling moribund when we experience the unwelcome, which, for us, includes stuttering. We refocus our outlook from considering ourselves as outsiders to seeing ourselves as part of the whole and by showing compassion to ourselves and to each other and become revitalized.

Tibetans practice *tonglen* to heal themselves when they are unwell. They visualize themselves taking on the discomfort of all who ail as they do. Then they extend wishes to all these beings and to themselves for well-being (e.g., Mipham, 2007). This practice can be used by anyone suffering for any reason (e.g., Lief, 2008; Chödrön, 2003b). We, for instance, can think of many others who have stuttering problems, children, teens, adults, men, women, residents of our country or residents of another place, and people who do not have stuttering problems but also feel misunderstood, alone, or rejected. Using breath as framework, we imagine ourselves taking on their suffering and sending them and ourselves wishes for well-being. This unconventional exchange of pleasant for unpleasant comprises the bulk of *tonglen* meditation practice. Practicing *tonglen*, we remember and reinforce the belief we are not alone in our pain. We are not outsiders.

When we feel angry because we fail to act as we wish, such as when we speak hardly at all to avoid stuttering, we can remember others, too, experience times when they disappoint themselves. *We are not the only one.* When we feel hurt when someone mocks us for stuttering, we can remember others, too, may be mocked for how they look or act. *We are not the only one.* When we feel sad because we believe we were turned down when asking someone out on a date because we stutter, we can remember others also feel hurt when someone they like rejects them. *We are not the only one.* When we are not offered the job we are seeking or the salary raise we are requesting, we can recall others, too, are not offered the jobs for which they apply or the raises they request. *We are not the only one.* And we can live this sense of solidarity by sending well-wishes to ourselves and to those suffering as we for happiness and for ease of being, as we do when we practice *maitri* (e.g., Salzberg, 2011). Doing so, our energy rises. We feel more present. We feel more purposeful. And we feel more willing to do what we need to do to change how we think and act to speak and live with greater ease.

Reminding ourselves of our solidarity with others, other people with stuttering problems and people without stuttering problems, dashes the notion we are separate and reinforces our understanding we are all fundamentally the same. By acknowledging we are not alone and that others, too, suffer as we do by sometimes feeling misunderstood, unappreciated, and rejected for seeming to be different, our sense of isolation fades. Yet, to be with others in good company can be daunting if we have lived in relative isolation for some time. We may feel unequipped or ill-equipped to socialize or to communicate effectively through speech at work and at home. So, we develop plans to acquire the knowledge and skills we need to communicate deftly and carry them out. And, just like everyone else we, too, will make mistakes learning to communicate skillfully. There will be times we will say things we wish we had not or not say things we wish we had said. There will be times we may be a little awkward making light conversation at parties or on dates. There will be times when we may not capture and hold our colleagues' attention as we would like at department meetings or share skillfully with our partners' during intimate conversation. And we may overlook the value of *smoozing*. But, like everyone else, we can gradually learn what we need to know and develop skill putting it into practice. We keep on keeping on, learning as we go. And, in the process, we develop a more balanced view of ourselves and experience increasing joy.

* * *

To consistently speak with greater ease requires us to strengthen our new beliefs and our new behaviors until they reliably replace older, stronger ones. Like other behaviors, unwanted speech and communication behaviors can persist even when the original need for them no longer exists. One such example surfaced several decades ago among children born with cleft palates. That was when surgeons in the United States waited until they were approximately four years-old to close the gaps in their palates, a procedure they and speech-language pathologists believed would automatically lead to clearer speech. Yet, some who experienced successful surgical repairs still required speech therapy to speak correctly despite a newly functional speech mechanism enabling them to direct speech sounds through their mouths. As they had been accustomed, many continued emitting speech sounds through their nasal cavities. That habit strength of only two or so years trumped the new functionality of their speech mechanism.

For those of us with stuttering problems who wish to change how we speak and communicate, we need to establish new beliefs and new behaviors to supplant learned ones we no longer wish to continue, a process which may be on-going for quite some time especially for those of us who began developing a stuttering problem as children. Releasing the fear and the fear-related behavior we feel when we stutter believing that, by stuttering, we may be rejected in some way, and incorporating into our daily life the willingness and skills to move out from the small space where we may be hiding from that fear to move more fully into our lives takes time and persistence. Mindfulness practice can help us skillfully cross over from living life our life as performance to living as our authentic selves while speaking with greater ease.

7

CHANGING

Things change. Plans change. Neighborhoods change. Nations change. They do not stay the same. Neither do we. We grow. We learn. We move on. And the way we think about stuttering and the way we stutter change too. How is up to us. We can continue fearing stuttering and struggling with stuttering trying to best it, and our current beliefs and behaviors will become more fixed. Or we can think and act differently to speak and live with greater ease. We have that choice. If we choose change, mindfulness can help. By being mindful, we become more alert to what we are thinking, feeling, and doing moment-by-moment and what is going on around us. This awareness prepares us to relate ever more skillfully to our stuttering by addressing fear as it arises and by becoming increasingly likely to respond skillfully rather than to react customarily. And we use two integral activities, *starting over* and *keeping going,* to strengthen our tendency to do so.

TWO INTEGRAL ACTIVITIES

When we begin to meditate, we may be surprised, even alarmed, at how difficult it can be for most of us to quiet and steady our mind, as a scene in the film *Eat Pray Love* well illustrates. We witness Julia Roberts, portraying writer Elizabeth Gilbert (2007), beginning what may be her first individual meditation session. She begins by sitting on the floor in tailor fashion, noting the time on the wall clock, and silently instructing herself to stop thinking. Then we witness her being distracted by an itch on her wrist, an insect landing on her neck, the revolving motion of the blades of the ceiling fan, and the apparent composure of a meditator sitting nearby. We hear her silently react to the experience with boredom, anxiety, and, finally, fierce self-recrimination as she observes herself allowing her mind to jump from thought to thought, judging, planning, and worrying. When she next looks at the clock, it is one minute later. Shocked and dismayed, she rises from the cushion and bolts for the door. During her agitated flight from the mediation room, she encounters an acquaintance, an experienced meditator, who acknowledges her distress and counsels her to continue practicing. He explains that she only will experience the peace she seeks if she learns to quiet her mind. A few weeks later, we see her sitting in silent meditation seemingly more focused. Perhaps, she is training her mind the way we might teach a puppy to stay by bringing it back and saying, "Stay," each time it wanders (Kornfield, 1996). We do not become angry with the puppy for wandering or impatient with the process for being repetitious. We matter-of-factly return the puppy to where we want him to be and gently, with kindness, repeat the command, "Stay" as many times as necessary. In this way, we train the puppy to stay. And so we can train our mind.

Starting Over

Because wandering is a well-known and common characteristic of the untrained mind, *starting over* is one of the very few instructions given those beginning the practice of *shamatha-vipassana* mindfulness mediation (e.g. Chödrön, 2005). These instructions are: 1) Relax, 2) Make yourselves comfortable, 3) Observe your breath, and 4) When your mind wanders, return your attention to your breath. At first, even though we know better, we may react to the need to start over with anger, annoyance, and shame because we think we have failed. After all, until we have tried meditating, we think that of all the things we have done and of all the things we need to do nothing could be easier than to relax, get comfortable, and attend to our breath. So, when we discover how challenging watching our breath can be, we can become stunned and discouraged. But, if we take a step back, we may come to recognize that starting over represents desirable growth: *We are becoming mindful enough to recognize when we have not been mindful.* And, by starting over, we are demonstrating our commitment to changing how we live. That is success, not failure. When we start over, we are saying we want to change, and we are. That is the true message of starting over.

One day, we may surprise ourselves by stopping and starting over as we drive, clean, shop, eat, bathe, participate in a tweet chat, or become involved with some other activity and notice our attention drift into or be ensnared by stories we are telling ourselves about a pleasant or painful memory, a regret, a fantasy, a concern, a need, or some other unresolved matter. As seamlessly, as when we are practicing *shamatha*, we withdraw our attention from these stories to return it to what we are doing. And, as we do, we can take a moment to acknowledge we are changing as we wish. We do so briefly because we do not want to distract ourselves with self-appreciation any more than we would want to waylay ourselves with self-deprecation. We are learning to prefer being quietly present in the moment. This is how we live more mindfully and become more comfortable.

Learning to successfully manage relapses into accustomed mindlessness while we meditate or as we engage in tasks and perform activities during daily life prepares us to skillfully manage relapses into avoiding stuttering. But, for many of us, relapse into struggling with stuttering brings a stronger sense of failure than relapse into accustomed mindlessness while meditating or when preparing dinner because we often carry with us a painful history associated with learning to change how we speak and the way we approach speaking. Once, or more than once, we may have chosen to follow a plan to change and did so until we inadvertently reverted to our accustomed patterns of avoidance and struggle in one or more circumstances. Then our limited, unhelpful understanding of relapse spooked us into mistakenly concluding that our bodies, the methods we were using, or both had betrayed us. Equating relapse with failure, we felt profound anger and hurt. We felt betrayed. We even may have feared we just could not change. Our renewed hope we could speak with greater ease seemed dashed. We felt bested by our stuttering yet again. And we felt weak, helpless, and, even, disheartened. From the depth of our being, we may have asked, "Why?" Finding no other answers, we may have decided we were physically incapable of speaking differently or we may have concluded the way we were going about changing was not right for us, so we withdrew from the program that seemingly failed us, becoming ever more convinced speaking with ease was not for us, at least not yet. When it might be, we did not know. So we carried on doing as we have done, strengthening accustomed patterns of belief and behavior, hoping we might change, uncertain whether we could, and suffering from an agony of uncertainty laced both with hope and doubt that generated general and focused anger toward ourselves and others for not remedying our sense of failure and isolation. This misinformed take on relapse helped grow our problem.

For many, this is our potent back story that encourages us to relate to relapse as a cue to quit. Recognizing that, we patiently apply our new understanding of relapse as encouragement to keep going instead.

Keeping Going

Sometimes we do not want to continue our practice. This happens. We tell ourselves we are too tired or too busy to sit for daily practice. We may feel bored with our practice or dissatisfied having to wait for results. Under these circumstances, we may be tempted to quit. We want the results we hoped for but not the discipline of the routine, which is like hoping to lose extra pounds without following a daily practice of eating less and moving more. We are forgetting we can not speak with greater ease without doing the necessary work (e.g., Kongtrül, 2006). Rather than forcing ourselves to do what we dislike and risk building further resentment toward our practice that could, in time, sabotage our chance of realizing our goal, we can explore alternates to the form of our current practice, since a critical feature of practice is experimentation (Salzberg, 2011; Nelson, 2010). We can, for instance, reduce the time we spend in practice. If 20 minutes is too much, we can spend 15, 10, or, even, 5 minutes daily in sitting meditation since some meditation is considered better than none at all (e.g., Salzberg, 2011; Mipham, 2006). We can practice mindfulness as we climb or descend flights of stairs, as we stir pancake batter, perform exercises with free weights, ride a stationary bike, or skip rope, actions we can perform slowly enough so we can attend to our breath as we do so. And we can switch, at least temporarily, to a motion-based practice. Walking mediation, for example (e.g., Salzberg, 2011; Brown, 2007; Hanh & Nyugen, 2006), a form of *shamatha*, or insight, meditation, increases our sensitivity to our body. Attending to the sensations involved with lifting then placing our feet during this practice increases our awareness of how we move, which we can transfer to how we position and move our jaw, tongue, and lips as we speak and anticipate speaking.

Although, there seems to be no substitute for sitting or moving meditation to become increasingly skillful at quieting and managing the mind and becoming sensitive to messages the body sends, *maitri, lojong, gatha*, and *tonglen* practices, which can be applied on-the-spot anywhere, can help highlight our commitment to becoming more mindful. So, too, can reading instructive books, listening to CD's, or watching DVD's introducing the rationale and practice of mindfulness, especially those by Pema Chödrön, Thich Nhat Hanh, Dzigar Kongtrül, Jack Kornfield, Sakyong Mipham, and Sharon Salzberg and reading magazines such as *Tricycle, Buddhadarma*, and *Shambhala Sun*. But it is primarily through ongoing practice that we learn to be increasingly effective at noticing and relating skillfully to our thoughts, emotions, and body sensations with kindness and compassion. Through practice, we not only enlarge our understanding of who we are we develop skills to live more consistently and comfortably as we genuinely are. Why forego this opportunity?

SPOTTING SIGNS OF CHANGE

There will come a time after we begin meditating when we wonder why we continue to do it. We do not feel more content with our lives. Nor do we feel stronger. In fact, we may not feel different at all. Then, unexpectedly, perhaps eight weeks or so from the time we began mindfulness meditation, we begin to notice positive changes in our behavior (e.g., Baime, 2011). We find ourself saying a kind word to a stranger maneuvering through the same crowded supermarket aisle as we. For a moment, we are stunned. We realize we were present enough to perceive her as another human being, someone like us also frustrated, rather than as we usually do, as an obstacle to getting what we want when we want it. At home, working on a fix-it project, we surprise ourself by working until we complete the task rather than escaping to play video games as we usually do when facing a temporarily daunting challenge. And when we began swearing after dropping a plate of spaghetti with red sauce on the kitchen floor, we uncharacteristically stop, recalling the saying, "Don't wallow in self-pity." We refuse to swear and flail about as we usually do knowing we would only deepen our anger, and we would still have to clean up the mess. These unplanned and unexpected changes come ". . . on little cat feet . . . " (Sandburg, 1916), quietly announcing in fundamental and desirable ways we are changing. We see we are instinctively applying to our everyday life what we are learning in *maitri, lojong, gatha,* and *tonglen* practices and through *shenpa* work. We are relating more mindfully and with greater wisdom and kindness to ourselves and others, as we do doing *shamatha-vipassana* practice, when we, otherwise, may have related harshly or been unaware.

As we continue to practice, we may begin to spot instances when we also relate more constructively to our actual stuttering or our concerns about our stuttering. These changes, too, may arise unexpectedly and quietly. For example, as we become fearful approaching the counter staff at a deli to order a meal, we uncharacteristically draw our attention away from our racing pulse to place it on the movement of our breath without judgment or comment and without the desire to control it as we do during *shamatha-vipassana*. Another time, rather than worrying how we might come across if we stutter as we enter a room to attend a reception, we unexpectedly choose to softly attend to the placement of our feet, the way we might during movement meditation, as we walk to the bar. And during a staff meeting, we might surprise ourself by silently offering wishes of well-being to a colleague as she presents and defends an unpopular but necessary plan for company debt-reduction rather than worry, as we usually do, whether we will be fluent when it is our turn to present. Unexpectedly applying attitudes and skills developed in mindfulness practices that smoothes our interactions with others tells us they are infiltrating our being. This is an unmistakable sign we are changing.

These traces of change excite us, but they can be dangerous, as poet Alexander Pope (1709) warned, ". . . a little knowledge is a dangerous thing. . ." Through them, we see we can relate more skillfully to our stuttering and our thoughts about stuttering to speak and live with greater ease. Acknowledging that, we feel more energetic. We feel more masterful than we have for some time. And we feel more hopeful we will speak and live as we wish and, possibly, soon. But, if we let this new-found excitement seduce us into stopping meditating because we think we now know how to apply mindfulness strategies to our stuttering problem, we can crash, reverting to longer-lived, less helpful ways of thinking about and relating to our stuttering when faced with formidable stress and fear. Although it may be eight weeks or more since we started this transformative practice, we have just begun to learn these skills and attitudes that can help carry us to where we want to be. Like someone learning to play the acoustic guitar who has learned just enough fingering to play a few basic chords and to do some elementary picking and strumming, we have learned only enough to know what we are learning during practice can be transferred to daily life and that we can do so. We need to continue meditation practice to hone and strengthen these emerging skills so they become malleable and durable enough for us to express ourselves as freely as we wish at will. If we remain committed to stuttering with greater ease by practicing mindfulness, we will continue mindfulness mediation practices. That also will help us manage the anger we may hold for having and having had a stuttering problem and the universal fears about changing we, too, may need to address (e.g., Myss, 1998).

ADDRESSING FEAR

Engaging in *vipassana*, we may discover that, although we believe we want to change, we may subconsciously fear what change may bring (e.g., Silverman, 2007). That is common and a reason why some do not heal (e.g,. Myss, 1998). Fear of change can appear in surprising ways. Fear can underlie our belief we are too busy to continue meditating or to start (e.g., Chödrön, 2011b; Gimian, 2010). Because, like most people we know, we *are* busy, we may not recognize this belief as more a statement of fear of change than an accurate assessment of our situation and, as such, a convenient excuse not to do what we need to do to change (Dyer, 2011). Letting go of unhelpful beliefs about ourselves, others, and the world we may be using as excuses can be difficult.

By the time we are adults, we have developed ideas about ourselves, others, and stuttering based on experiences we have had primarily as children and teens that, unchecked, govern our lives as adults (e.g, Berne, 1996; Steiner, 1994; Woollums and Brown, 1979). A few, such as the importance of being heard, can help us live more openly and fully. Some, which depend on others' opinions of us as much as or more than our own, may lead to a claustrophobic, stifled existence. Beliefs are like that. They lead us to act and, by so doing, fashion our present circumstances. Unless and until we recognize them and update them based on our more extensive knowledge and experience, living out beliefs developed when we were young can short-change our experience of life and lead to us to feel stuck.

We often erroneously assume our beliefs are us, and we fear by discarding them we will compromise our identity and become unknown even to ours own eyes (e.g., Steiner, 1994). But beliefs are just beliefs. They are mental positions (e.g., Tolle, 2005). They are not who we are (e.g., Crick, 1994; Whitney, 1985). They are conclusions we have reached about ourselves, others, and stuttering when we were children and teens and less experienced and capable of analytic reasoning (e.g., Berne, 1996; Steiner, 1994). Continuing to heed them, leads us to function primarily as conveyances for our young selves, who, metaphorically, perch on our shoulders calling the shots and tell us when, where, and with whom we should speak. Perhaps, for this reason, psychoanalyst Carl Jung reportedly believed, "We do not solve our problems. We outgrow them. We grow up" (Dyer, 2011). Growing up is considered the great fruit, or realization of mindfulness practice according to Chöygam Trungpa Rinpoche (Chödrön, 2009).

Mindfulness is a tool we can use to free ourselves from this self-imposed tyranny (e.g., Chödrön, 2011b) the way Michelangelo sculpted stone. He hewed away elements that obscured the figure he saw within. He did not sculpt lions or horses or David's. He removed parts of the block of stone that were not a lion or a horse or the legendary warrior, then polished the figure that remained. The process can be lengthy and challenging. For instance, the sculptor of the Crazy Horse Memorial, Korcazk Ziólkowski, who used dynamite to reveal his vision of the noted American Indian leader within the Black Hills Mountains of South Dakota, began the still unfinished monument in 1948.

The process of release and refinement characterizes the activity of all who seek to become whole (e.g., von Franz, 1964), which echoes the process of polishing a beach stone by tumbling it with grit. As Zen Master Shunryo Suzuki Roshi told an audience gathered to hear him speak at the San Francisco Zen Center (Chödrön, (2005), "You are all perfect, and you can use a little work," suggesting we all may be diamonds in the rough. Similarly, Carl Jung believed we do not need to become someone else to live as we wish; we only need to release what obstructs us from doing so and then do so wholeheartedly (e.g., Whitney, 1985; van Franz, 1964). For many of us with stuttering problems, who shied away from opportunities to talk for most of our lives, that can include cultivating undeveloped or underdeveloped communication skills, such as those we can use to make small talk with family, friends, acquaintances, co-workers, and strangers as well as those to converse with ease, interview ably, negotiate satisfactorily in personal and work-related matters, argue skillfully, speak effectively before a group, and so forth.

Practitioners of various psychotherapies, such as Transactional Analysis (e.g., Berne, 1996) and Mindfulness Based Cognitive Therapy (MBCT) (e.g., Segal, *et al.*, 2002), as well as adherents of the linguistic based theory of human change, General Semantics (e.g., Johnson, 1980; Korzybski, 1955), share Jung's belief. They also share his unwillingness to view those of us who feel stuck in our lives as broken needing to be fixed. They view us as traversing a stage of growth that includes freeing ourselves from a confining fear of change (e.g., Whitney, 1985; von Franz, 1964) and themselves as personal educators offering information, direction, and support.

Using mindfulness to free ourselves, like using dynamite to sculpt a form from a mountainside, can bring forth a seismic event. We can be rocked as we recognize who our work exposes. It is we who emerge, not someone who produces mechanically flawless speech, not someone whose sensibilities differ from our own, not someone different from us at all. It is we who surface, more present, more self-accepting, and more comfortable. If we stutter, we do so with aplomb. We have learned to focus on communicating, not performing. Like a beach stone transformed by tumbling in grit into a jewel-like object or a rough diamond converted by grinding and faceting into a gemstone, we now glisten.

The demolition work beginning with *shamatha-vipassana* removes our fear of stuttering like a nutcracker cracks the shell encasing a nut. Removing resistance to and struggle with fear from the way we stutter, we stutter fearlessly. We are learning what we did not know when we began fearing stuttering: *Stuttering can neither kill us nor brand us alien.* We can stutter and live, and we can stutter and belong. By renouncing our fear of stuttering, we no longer resist stuttering. We no longer respond to stuttering with silence and struggle nor hold to feelings of anger induced by fear. We recognize these reactions as diversions from constructive action. And we choose to communicate instead. As we do, we release our stuttering problem, *but not all at once* (e.g., Silverman, 2003).

Sometimes, though, it is not change we fear but the possibility we can not change. We can develop this belief when our attempts to change as children, teens, and, even, adults failed to meet expectations. Having thought we failed ourselves and, perhaps, those who cared for and about us or that these important people in our lives failed us and, now, we are too old, we may conclude we are destined to be undesirably different. The anger that belief arouses can mask our fear that change is not possible for us. And, rather than face that fear directly, we may find it easier to become angry believing life has given us a burden we can not jettison for reasons we can not fathom. Believing life is unfair can lead to being cynical, expecting the worst for ourselves and believing the worst of others. We may deplore others for seeming to be callous or indifferent to our pain of alienation. We may withdraw. Or we may become argumentative with those who suggest that the change we desire can be possible for us or for others like us, even abrasive, to spare ourselves the pain of more disappointment. Holding to these feelings of anger and the fearful beliefs underlying them, we may become reluctant to make a genuine effort to change, and, if we do, we may be impatient to see results and poised to quit if we do not see them as quickly as we wish and exactly as we wish.

We may feel stuck. But we are not. We think we are because we do not see the changes we want as quickly as we want to see them. To motivate ourselves to continue, we can think of ourselves as a lake or a river in winter. Although the surface may become ice, the entire body rarely does. Water continues to flow beneath the ice, sometimes only as a trickle, but it moves nonetheless.

RESPONDING NOT REACTING

Until we have been practicing mindfulness for some time, which can vary from person to person, we may feel angry and fearful much of the time. We may be angry with our stuttering, with ourselves for stuttering, with therapists who did not help us, with people seemingly insensitive or callous to our struggle to fit in, and with so-called society for limiting our opportunities to enjoy a more content life. And we still may fear stuttering itself and the possibility of stuttering because we dread feeling out-of-control. We generally come to accept these reactive responses as inevitable. But they are not. They are learned responses to stuttering that perpetuate our problem by shrinking our experience of life and reducing our opportunity to develop communication skills that can increase our enjoyment of life (e.g., Johnson, 1954). The longer we practice mindfulness, the more readily we recognize them and the more skilled we become at neutralizing these mindless reactions to our stuttering that fuel our problem by responding rather than reacting.

* * *

Establishing a personal mindfulness practice and settling into it can help us get from where we are to where we want to be. We start by allotting time, preferably the same time daily, for practice and, perhaps, additional time weekly to read books and magazine articles about developing and maintaining a practice as well as listen to CD's and podcasts and watch DVD's. But we do not let reading about meditating or listening to advice for building a practice substitute for practice itself. We know it is only through practice that we strengthen our awareness of what we are thinking, feeling, and doing in the moment and develop and hone the skills and attitudes to relate skillfully to our thoughts, emotions, and body sensations as they arise. Mindfulness meditation provides experience developing these skills in the presence of external distractions, such as sounds, scents, temperature, and other peoples' energies (e.g., Orloff, 2005; Leadbetter, 1977), and to internal distractions, such as worry, regret, impatience, boredom, physical discomfort, and so on, preparing us for applying them in ordinary life where distractions abound.

Practice resembles life. And, when we practice, we may be more deeply involved with life than otherwise. In practice, we determine to stay with what we dislike (e. g., Chödrön, 2011b; 2005). We get to know and accept our life as it is in the moment, and, as we do, ourselves as well. What we think and feel as we practice during sitting or moving meditation is the same as what we think and feel at other times. When we meditate, we feel emotions, large and small, such as anger, fear, resentment, and disappointment, aversion, and bitterness; we feel tension, tightness, throbbing, and other body sensations; and we feel the urge to be somewhere else and the desire to do something else. By meditating and engaging in the supplemental mindfulness practices of *maitri, tonglen, lojong,* and the recitiation of *gathas* we learn to notice and to accept our thoughts, emotions, and bodily sensations as they arise and to relate kindly and skillfully to them, to ourselves, and, ultimately, to others. We learn we are not our thoughts, no more than we are our emotions. We understand nothing is permanent, including our emotions, body sensations, and circumstances. And we recognize we are not the only one who suffers from feeling misunderstood or rejected. We apply this awareness to our fear of stuttering, our anger about stuttering, our regret for stuttering, our shame for stuttering, our desire to avoid stuttering, and our stuttering itself.

How long it may take to journey to where we want to be can not be predicted for us individually or collectively at this time, if ever. Few of us, may take a straight trajectory or the same trajectory. The trek by nature is individual. We may seem to go forward, pause, backtrack, then move forward, and repeat the process. Occasionally we may move sideways. Until we complete the journey, we may not know with certainty the trajectory we are following (e.g., von Franz, 1964). So we suspend judgment about how well we are doing and how far we have come and simply attend to meditating and living mindfully in the moment with the confidence that, if we do, we will experience change we desire.

We organize our life around meeting our responsibilities with kindness and care and following our curiosity. This may lead to new interests and hobbies, such as drawing and painting, black and white photography, singing in a group, meatless cooking, cycling, walking, mouth blowing glass, journaling, practicing the martial art of *ninpo*, gardening with native plants, studying alchemy and mysticism, and so on, all with the intent of expanding and strengthening our experience of living mindfully. Our path also may include enrolling in speech therapy or counseling for information and coaching to help us change. If so, we will benefit most if we decide beforehand specifically what we want to relate about our experience and what we want to learn (e.g., Charon, 2008; Woolams and Brown, 1979), just as we do when we sign

up for an enrichment course, which is what therapy and counseling essentially can be (e.g., Whitney, 1985).

This is not to suggest we will enjoy every moment of the journey. We will not. We can encounter truths about ourselves, often
while performing the most mundane tasks, such as taking out the
garbage, which we would rather keep buried. Such discoveries
may be more challenging to address than our stuttering itself.
We may feel great pain, shame, guilt, and even anger with ourselves when we realize we have thought and acted in ways that
twisted us and may have hurt others at times. But we do not
cling to these emotions of shame and regret. We realize doing
so harms us and can disturb others (e.g., Myss, 1998). We feel,
observe, and examine them as deftly and as fully as we can, then
release them, resolving never again to knowingly harm ourselves
or another in that way now that we know better (e.g., Salzberg,
2011; Chödrön, 2005; Kornfield, 1996). To change, we do not
need to know why we thought or acted as we did. We change by
changing (e.g., Kongtrül, 2006; Berne, 1996).

Sometimes, we may recall being hurt by another. I have not
known a person whether they have a stuttering problem or not
who has not felt hurt by the intentional or unintentional words or
actions of another. During meditation, perhaps, for the first time
in years, we who have stuttering problems may re-experience
the pain, shame, and, perhaps, the horror we believe someone's
behavior brought us. We may recall the bullying, the taunting,
the callous laughter, the dismissive comments, and the awkward
silence that encouraged us to feel as an alien. We recall, too,
the words and deeds of parents, teachers, and therapists trying
to help us change that encouraged us to feel we were not good
enough.

We remember those times, touching them lightly with our
attention. We do not brush these memories away. Realizing we
now are in a safer place, we stay with the emotions that arise

from these remembrances. We allow ourselves to feel them as carefully and as fully as we can then we release them as we would a distracting thought that arises during *shamatha-vipas-sana* practice. We do not hold onto such remembrances. No healing can come from that. But healing can come from silently offering forgiveness when we are ready to those whose words or actions hurt us, including ourselves. Our practice of *maitri* can help (e.g., Salzberg, 2011; 2005). We release the anger we hold, the desire we may have for revenge, and the shame we may feel. We do this primarily for our own sakes. We know holding onto anger and living in shame harms us (e.g., Kornfield, 1996; Weil, 1995). We choose to be well. We move on.

Subject Index

A

absent-minded 21-23

anger 16, 24, 25, 30, 38, 39,
42, 42, 46, 55, 63, 67, 68,
87, 90- 91, 97, 102, 107,
115, 121, 124-125, 127-128

Asanas 29

avoidance 42- 43, 52, 54, 62,
71, 116

awareness 18, 21, 25, 36, 45,
51, 52, 56, 64, 84, 101,
108, 113, 118, 126-127,
153-154, 160

B

brain 5, 7, 14, 18, 37, 40-41,
145, 148, 153

breath 9-10, 15, 24, 29-30,
36-37, 39-40, 45, 56-59,
66-68, 86, 102-103, 106,
109, 115, 117, 119, 137, 147

Buddhism 4, 24, 146

Buddhist 3-5, 9, 62, 74, 85,
92, 94, 104, 138-140, 143-
144, 147, 155, 159

C

Calming the Mind 35

Centering Prayer 5, 11

change 6-9, 11, 14-19, 23-26,
30-31, 35-36, 40-41, 43,
46, 49-51, 53-55, 58-59,
61, 63, 65, 71, 76-77, 79,
84, 88, 91, 93-96, 99-100,
103, 106, 111, 113, 116,
119-121, 123, 125, 127,
129, 137, 140, 144, 147,
149

control 31, 57, 64, 72, 97,
102-103, 119, 148

D

denial 22, 54, 84

distracted 21-24, 29, 34, 37,
39, 58, 114

distracted mind 24

E

ease 2, 4-5, 9, 11, 24-25,
32, 35-36, 38, 40, 45-46,
49-53, 56, 58, 60-65, 68,

70, 72-74, 76-77, 79-81,
84-85, 88-96, 9-106, 110-
111, 113, 116-117, 120-23,
157, 159
Empiricists 116
Equanimity 139, 157

F
fear 2, 3, 18, 31-33, 38-39,
41-47, 4, 51, 54, 61-63, 65,
67-70, 90-91, 97-99, 106-
107, 111, 113, 120-127,
139 141, 146, 155

G
Gatha's 80, 101-102
General Semantics 89, 123,
143, 145
getting unstuck 63-64, 139

H
Happiness 15, 51, 84-85, 87,
101-102, 106-107, 110,
138 142, 147, 155
Hooked 4, 140, 159,

I
Insight Meditation 3, 6, 36, 39,
68, 118, 147-148, 153

J
Jewish scriptures 4

K
kindness 16, 26, 53, 75,
80-83, 86, 90, 114, 118-
119, 127, 147
Koan 100

L
Logotherapist 97
Lojong 3-4, 80, 91-92, 94,
108, 118-119, 126, 139, 59
Looking and Seeing 35, 37
Lovingkindness 82, 138

M
Maitri 3, 4, 79-80, 82, 84, 85,
92, 100, 110, 118-119, 127,
129, 159
Meditation 1, 3-11, 14, 16-17,
19, 29, 31-40, 44-45, 47,
49, 50-55, 57, 59, 62-64,
68, 70, 73, 80, 84, 94, 102-
104, 108-109, 114, 117-
118, 120, 126, 129, 138,
140, 143, 145-149, 153,
156, 159
Metta 80, 147
Mindfulness 1, 2, 4-5, 10,
13, 16-18, 21, 24, 29,
33,35, 45, 49, 51-52, 77,
79, 111, 113, 115, 118, 122,
125-126, 137-138, 142-
145, 148-150, 153, 155,
157, 159-160

Mindfulness Based Cognitive Therapy (MBCT 123. 148
Mindfulness Based Stress Reduction (MBSR) 26
Mindfulness Meditation Practice 3, 5, 7, 16, 35, 38, 47, 102
monkey mind 35
moving meditation 118, 126

N
Negative Self-Talk 30, 31
Neuroplasticity 12-14
Neuroscience 7, 153

O
openness 30, 34, 91

P
Paradoxical Intention 54, 62, 97
paying attention 9
performance 50, 111
practice 1, 4-11, 14-16, 24, 35, 37, 40, 49-50, 53, 56, 71, 79, 117, 138-140, 142-147, 150, 157, 160
Pranayama 102-103, 147
present 3, 17-19, 26, 35, 54, 57, 63, 116, 143, 150

R
Rationalists 16

Recognizing 62, 64, 108
relapse 53, 116-117
relax 9, 23, 32, 47, 52, 70-71, 73, 86, 90, 94, 115
Relaxing 23, 62, 69-70
Renouncing 62, 65, 67-68, 124
resistance 41 61, 64, 67, 70-71, 75, 94, 124
responding 54, 65, 67, 125
resolving 67, 71, 128

S
self-help 10, 14, 97
self-mastery 11, 30-32 34
sensations 3, 7, 14, 34, 33-40, 42-45, 47, 52, 56, 63-68, 70, 74, 94, 106, 118, 126-127
Shamatha 35, 53-55, 60, 101, 115, 118, 146
Shamatha-Vipassana 3, 6, 7, 30, 33, 36, 52, 55, 80, 85, 94, 103, 115, 119, 124, 129, 156, 159
Shenpa 2-4, 23, 33, 41-42, 44, 49, 52-53, 61-64, 70, 73, 75-76, 80, 84-85, 119, 149, 159
sitting meditation 62, 117, 156
slogans 91-93, 101
Speech Pathologists 77, 88-89, 157

Speech Therapy 85, 105, 111, 127

Spirit Rock Meditation Center 6, 153

Staying 3, 36, 41, 43-44, 54, 61-62

Stopping and Looking 55

struggle 3, 38, 42, 46, 54, 57-58, 65-66, 68-69, 71, 85, 94, 99, 116, 124

stuttering 2, 4-5, 7-10 13, 17-18, 23, 25, 32-33, 38, 40, 42, 49, 52, 59, 62, 64-65, 69, 83, 86, 88, 98, 107, 110, 113, 121, 125, 137-138, 140-144, 148-151, 154-155, 157, 159-160

suffering 15, 55, 66, 104, 107-108, 110

T

The Age of Reason 15

The Insight Meditation Society 6

Tibetan 2, 4, 41, 62, 85, 92, 109, 140, 159

Tonglen 3-4, 80, 104, 108-109, 118-119, 126, 140, 145, 159

Transactional Analysis 89, 123, 137, 150-151, 159

U

unconditional friendship 75

V

Vipassana 3-4, 6-7, 30, 33, 36-37, 52-56, 60, 68, 76, 80, 84-86, 89, 94, 102-106, 115, 119, 121, 124, 129, 156, 159

W

welcome 44, 54, 67, 70, 75, 98

Welcoming Prayer 5

well-wishing 81, 83-84

Z

Zen 5, 24, 36, 50, 100, 122-123, 145, 155

References

Allione, T., (2008). *Feeding Your Demons. Ancient Wisdom for Solving Inner Conflict.* New York: Little, Brown and Company.

Altman, D. (2011). *One Minute Mindfulness.* Novato, California: New World Library.

Baime, M. (2011). "This is your brain on mindfulness." *Shambhala Sun,* July, 44-48; 84-85.

Balakrishnan, J., (2009). *Yoga for Stuttering: Unifying the Voice, Breath, Mind, and Body to Achieve Fluent Speech.* Berkeley, California: North Atlantic Books.

Barrows, A. and Macy, J. (1996), (Translators). *Rilke's Book of Hours: Love Poems to God.* New York: Riverhead.

Beckwith, L. (2008). *A Shine of Rainbows.* Cornwall, UK: House of Stratus.

Begley, S. (2010). "Forget the cocaine vaccine. Low-tech treatments work better." *Newsweek,* March 14, p 20.

Begley, S. (2007). *Train Your Mind, Change Your Brain: How a New Science Reveals Our Extraordinary Potential to Transform Ourselves.* New York: Ballantine Books.

Berne, E. (1996). *Games People Play. The Basic Handbook of Transactional Analysis.* New York: Ballantine, Re-Issue Edition.

Biden, J. (2009). " Vice President Joe Biden receives the 'Annie.'" *The ASHA LEADER,* Vol., 14, (16), p. 19.

Bloodstein, O. (1969). *A Handbook on Stuttering.* Chicago: National Easter Seal Society for Crippled Children and Adults.

Boorstein, S., Hollander, J., Brussat, F., and Brussat, M.A. (2010). *Lovingkindness with Sylvia Boorstein: An Online Retreat and Practice Circle.* New York: Spirituality & Practice.

Boorstein, S. (2008). *Happiness is an Inside Job: Practicing for a Joyful Life.* New York: Ballantine Books.

Boorstein, S. (1998). *That's Funny. You Don't Look Buddhist: On Being a Faithful Jew and a Passionate Buddhist.* New York: HarperCollins.

Boyce, B., (2011). *The Mindfulness Revolution. Leading Psychologists, Scientists, Artists, and Meditation Teachers on the Power of Mindfulness In Daily Life.* Boston: Shambhala Publications.

Boyce, B., (2010). "Why we're taking mindfulness to heart." *Shambhala Sun,* March, p. 11.

Brown, E. (2010). "Let your passion cook." *Shambhala Sun,* March, pp. 38-41.

Brown, E. (2007). *How to Cook Your Life.* New York: Lionsgate. (DVD)

Charon, R. (2008). *Narrative Medicine: Honoring the Stories of Illness.* New York: Oxford University Press-USA.

Carroll, M. (2010). "Beyond the elevator speech." *Shambhala Sun,* March, pp. 54-57.

Campbell, J. (1998). *Sukhavati – Place of Bliss; A Mythic Journey with Joseph Campbell*. Williston, VT: Mystic Fire Video. (DVD)

Chödrön, P. (2011b). *Smile at Fear: A Retreat with Pema Chödrön on Discovering Your Radiant Self-Confidence*. Boston: Shambhala Audio. (CD's)

Chödrön, P. (2011a). *Be Grateful to Everyone. An In-Depth Guide to the Practice of Lojong*. Boston: Shambhala Audio. (7 CD's)

Chödrön, P. (2010). *The Wisdom of No Escape: And the Path of Loving-Kindness*. Boston: Shambhala Publications.

Chödrön, P. (2009). *Perfect Just As You Are: Buddhist Practices on the Four Limitless Ones – Loving-Kindness, Compassion, Joy, and Equanimity*. Boston: Shambhala Audio. (Audio CD)

Chödrön, P. (2008). In S. Meyerowitz, (Director), *Teachings on Milarepa*. San Jose, California: Cinequest, Inc. (DVD)

Chödrön, P. (2007). *Always Maintain a Joyful Mind: And Other Lojong Teachings on Awakening Compassion and Fearlessness*. Boston: Shambhala Publications. (Includes Audio CD)

Chödrön, P. (2005). *Getting Unstuck*. Boulder, Colorado: Sounds True. (Audio CD)

Chödrön, P. (2005). *Practicing Peace in Times of War*. Boston: Shambhala Publications, Inc. (Audio CD)

Chödrön, P. (2004b). *Start Where You Are. A Guide to Compassionate Living*. Boston: Shambhala Publications.

Chödrön, P. (2004a). *Perfect Meditation*. Boulder, Colorado: Sounds True. (Audio CD).

Chödrön, P. (2003b). *Meditation for Difficult Times. Awakening Compassion Through The Practice of Tonglen*. Boulder, Colorado: Sounds True. (Audio CD)

Chödrön, P. (2003a). "How we get hooked/How to get unhooked." *Shambhala Sun*, March, pp. 30-35.

Conture, E. (2000). *Stuttering: Its Nature, Diagnosis, and Treatment,* 3rd Edition. Boston: Allyn & Bacon.

Crick, F. (1994). The Astonishing Hypothesis. The Scientific Search for the Soul. New York: Charles Scribners Sons.

Das, S. (1997). *Awakening the Buddha Within*. New York: Bantam Books.

Davidson, R., and Harrington, A. (Eds.) (2001). *Visions of Compassion: Western Scientists and Tibetan Buddhists Examine Human Nature*. Oxford, United Kingdom: Oxford University Press.

Didion, J. (2007). *The Year of Magical Thinking*. New York: Vintage.

Dyer, W. (2011). *Excuses Be Gone*. Carlsbad, California: Hay House. (DVD)

Dyer, W. (2009). *Change Your Thoughts – Change Your Life: Living the Wisdom of the Tao*. Carlsbad, California: Hay House. (DVD)

Edwards, B. (1999). *The New Drawing on the Right Side of the Brain: A Course in Enhancing Creativity and Artistic Confidence*. New York: Jeremy Tarcher.

Eliot, T. S. (1962). *The Wasteland.* New York: Harcourt.

Ellis, A. and Harper, R. (1975). *A Guide to Rational Living*, 3rd Edition. Chatsworth, California: Wilshire Book Company.

Fehmi, L. and Robbins, J. (2007). *The Open-Focus Brain. Harnessing the Power Of Attention to Heal Mind and Body.* Boston: Trumpeter.

Fischer, N. (2010). "Getting started." *Shambhala Sun*, September, 48-49; 75-76.

Frankl, V. (1959). *Man's Search for Meaning.* New York: Simon & Schuster.

Fraser, M. (1989). *Self-Therapy for the Stutterer, 7th Edition.* Memphis: Stuttering Foundation of America.

Fusco, K. (2004). *Tending to Grace.* New York: Knopf Books.

Geller, S. & Greenberg, L. (2012). *Therapeutic Presence: A Mindful Approach to Effective Therapy.* Washington, D.C.: American Psychological Association.

Gilbert, E. (2007). *Eat, Pray, Love: One Woman's Search for Everything Through Italy, India, and Indonesia.* New York: Penguin.

Gimian, C., Ed. (2010). *Smile at Fear: Awakening the Heart of Bravery.* Boston: Shambhala Publications.

Goffman, E. (1959). *Presentation of Self in Everyday Life.* New York: Doubleday Anchor Books.

Goleman, D. (2010). "Making the right choice." *Shambhala Sun*, March, 58-61.

Goleman, D. (2006). *Social Intelligence. The New Science of Human Relationships.* New York: Bantam Greco, L. &

Hayes, S. (2008). *Acceptance & Mindfulness Treatments for Children & Adolescents: A Practitioner's Guide.* Oakland, California; New Harbinger Books.

Greenland, S. (2010). "Mindfulness for children." *Insight Journal*, Winter, pp. 25-29.

Guitar, B., (2005). *Stuttering: An Integrated Approach to Its Nature and Treatment.* Baltimore: Lippincott Williams & Wilkins.

H.H. the Dalai Lama, (2006). *How to See YOURSELF As You Really Are.* New York: Atria Books.

H.H. the Dalai Lama (2005). *The Universe in a Single Atom: The Convergence of Science and Spirituality.* New York: Broadway Books.

Hanh, T. N. (2011b). *Planting Seeds. Practicing Mindfulness with Children.* Berkeley, California: Parallax Press. (Includes a CD)

Hanh, T. N. (2011a). *One Buddha is Not Enough. A Story of Collective Awakening.* Berkeley, California. Parallax Press.

Hanh, T. N. (2010b). *Reconciliation: Healing the Inner Child.* Berkeley, California: Parallax Press.

Hanh, T. N. (2010a). *A Pebble for Your Pocket.* Berkeley, California: Plum Blossom Books.

Hanh, T. N. (2009). *Happiness: Essential Mindfulness Practices.* Berkely: Parallax Press.

Hanh, T. N. (2006b). *Mindfulness and Psychotherapy.* Boulder, Colorado: Sounds True, Inc. (Audio CD's)

Hanh, T. N. (2006a). *Present Moment Wonderful Moment: Mindfulness Verses for Daily Living*, 2nd Edition. Berkeley, California: Parallax Press.

Hanh, T. N. (2005). The Ultimate Dimension. Boulder, Colorado: Sounds True, Inc. (Audio CD's).

Hanh, T. N. (2003). *The Present Moment. A Retreat on the Practice of Mindfulness.* Boulder, Colorado: Sounds True, Inc. (CD's)

Hanh, T. N. (2002). *Be Free Where You Are.* Berkeley, California: Parallax Press.

Hanh, T. N. (1999). *The Heart of the Buddha's Teaching.* New York: Broadway Books.

Hanh, T.N. & Nguyen, A.-H. (2006). *Walking Meditation.* Boulder, Colorado: Sounds True, Inc. (Includes DVD & CD-ROM).

Harris, T. (2004). *I'm OK --- You're OK.* New York: Harper Paperbacks.

Hellman, L. (1973). *Pentimento: A Book of Portraits.* New York: Little, Brown, and Company.

Hopkins, J., (2008). *A Truthful Heart. Buddhist Practices for Connecting with Others.* Ithaca, N.Y.: Snow Lion Publications.

Johnson, W. (1980). *People in Quandries. The Semantics of Personal Adjustment.* San Francisco: International Society for General Semantics.

Johnson, W. (1956). "Stuttering," pp. 216-217. In W. Johnson, *et al.* (Ed.), *Speech Handicapped School Children, 2nd Edition.* New York: Harper & Brothers.

Jung, G. G. (1976). *Psychological Types. Collected Works of C.G. Jung, Vol. 6.* Princeton, N. J.: Princeton University Press.

Kabat-Zinn, J. (2005). *Coming to Our Senses: Healing Ourselves and The World Through Mindfulness.* New York: Hyperion.

Kamenetz, R. (2007). *The Jew in the Lotus: A Poet's Rediscovery of Jewish Identity in Buddhist India.* New York: HarperOne.

Kang, C., Riazuddin, S., Mondorf, J., Krasnevich, D., Friedman, P. Mullitkin, J., And Drayna, D. (2010). "Mutations in the lysosomal enzyme --- Targeting pathway and persistent stuttering." The New England Journal of Medicine, www.nejm.org February 10, 2010 (10.1056/NEJMoa0902630).

Katie, B. (2003). *Loving What Is: Four Questions That Can Change Your Life.* New York: Three Rivers Press.

Keating, T. (2002). *Open Mind, Open Heart: The Contemplative Dimension of the Gospel.* New York: Continuum International Publishing Group.

Kongtrül, D. (2008). *Light Comes Through: Buddhist Teaching on Awakening to Our Natural Intelligence.* Boston: Shambhala Publications.

Kongtrül, D. (2006). *It's Up to You. The Practice of Self-Reflection on the Buddhist Path.* Boston: Shambhala Publications.

Kornfield, J. (2009). *The Wise Heart. A Guide to the Universal Teachings of Buddhist Psychology.* New York: Bantam.

Kornfield, J. (2005). *Meditation for Beginners.* Boulder, Colorado: Sounds True. (DVD).

Kornfield, J. (1996). *The Inner Art of Mediation.* Boulder, Colorado: Sounds True. (VHS Video)

Korzybski, A. (1955). *Science and Sanity, 5th Edition.* Fort Worth, Texas: Institute of General Semantics.

Kubler-Ross, E. (1997). *On Death and Dying.* New York: Scribners.

Landin, B. (2008). "Meditation can alter brain function and reduce stress." www.timesonline.co.uk/tol/life_and_style/health/article3554215.ece.

Langer, E. (1990). *Mindfulness.* New York: Da Capo Press.

Leadbetter, C.W. (1977). *The Chakras.* Wheaton, Ill.: Quest Books. 75-76.

Lief, J. (2008). "Tonglen. The Practice of Transformation," pp. 65-80. In S. Piver (Ed.), *Quiet Mind: A Beginner's Guide to Meditation.* Boston: Shambhala Publications. (Includes a CD)

Loori, J. D. (2008). *Bringing the Sacred to Life: The Daily Practice of Zen Ritual.* Boston: Shambhala Publications.

Mayberg, H., Silva, J., Brannan, J.,Tekell,J., Mahurun,R., McGinnis, S., and Jerabek, P., (2002). "The functional neuroanatomy of the placebo effect." *American Journal of Psychiatry*, 159, May, 728-737.

Mipham, S. (2010). "Peace in the fast lane." *Shambhala Sun*, January, pp. 19-21.

Mipham, S. (2009). How will I use this day? *Shambhala Sun*, March, pp. 17-18; 21.

Mipham, S. (2008). "Shamatha. The Practice of Tranquility," pp. 1-30. In S. Piver (Ed.), *Quiet Mind: A Beginner's Guide to Meditation*. Boston: Shambhala Publications. (Includes a CD)

Mipham, S. (2007). *Ruling Your World. Ancient Strategies for Modern Life: A Workshop*. Boston: Shambhala Audio. (CD's).

Mipham, S. (2006). *Ruling Your World. Ancient Strategies for Modern Life*. New York: Morgan Road Books.

Myers, I. (1995). *Gifts Differing: Understanding Personality Type*, 2nd Edition. Boston: Nicholas Brealey Publishing.

Myss, C. (2002). *Spiritual Madness: The Necessity of Meeting God in Darkness*. Boulder: Sounds True, Inc. (CD)

Myss, C. (1998). *Why People Don't Heal and How They Can*. New York: Three Rivers Press.

Nelson, J. (2010). "Experimental Buddhism." *Tricycle*. Winter, pp. 46-47; 111.

Orloff, J. (2005). *Positive Energy. Ten Extraordinary Prescriptions for Transforming Fatigue, Stress, and Fear into Vibrance, Strength, and Love*. New York: Three Rivers Press.

Pope, A. (1709). *An Essay on Criticism*. Memphis, Tennessee: General Books, LLC.

Piver, S. (Ed.) (2008). *Quiet Mind: A Beginner's Guide to Meditation. Six Simple Practices Presented by Leading*

Buddhist Teachers. Boston: Shambhala Publications. (Includes CD)

Ponlop, D. (2010). *Rebel Buddha. On the Road to Freedom.* Boston: Shambhala Publications.

Ray, R. (2008). *Touching Enlightenment. Finding Realization in the Body.*Boulder, Colorado: Sounds True, Inc.

Rosen, R. (2010). *The Practice of Pranayama. An In-Depth Guide to the Yoga of Breath.* Boston: Shambhala Audio. (CD's)

Rosenberg, L. (2008). "Vipasanna. The Practice of Clear Seeing," pp.31-42. In S. Piver, (Ed.), *Quiet Mind. A Beginner's Guide to Meditation. Six Simple Practices Presented by Leading Buddhist Teachers.* Boston: Shambhala Publications. (Includes a CD).

Salzberg, S. (2011). *Real Happiness. The Power of Mediation. A 28-Day Program.* New York: Workman Publishers. (Includes a CD) Salzberg, S. (2008). "Metta. The Practice of Compassion," pp. 53-64. In S. Piver (Ed.), *Quiet Mind: A Beginner's Guide to Meditation.* Boston: Shambhala Publications. (Includes a CD)

Salzberg, S., (2005). *The Force of Kindness: Change Your Life with Love and Compassion.* Boulder, Colorado: Sounds True, Inc. (CD's)

Salzberg, S. (1999). *A Heart as Wide as the World.* Boston: Shambhala Publications.

Salzberg, S. (1996). *Loving Kindness Meditation. Learning to Love through Insight Meditation.* Boulder, Colorado: Sounds True, Inc. (Audio CD's)

Salzberg, S. and Goldstein, J. (2004). *Insight Meditation.* Boulder, Colorado: Sounds True, Inc. (Includes CD)

Sandburg, C. (1916). *Chicago Poems.* Memphis, Tennessee: General Books, LLC.

Schwartz, J. and Gladding, R. (2011). *You Are Not Your Brain. The 4-Step Solution for Ending Bad Habits, Ending Unhealthy Thinking, and Taking Control of Your Life.* New York: Avery.

Segal, Z., Teasdale, J., Williams, M. (2002). *Mindfulness-Based Cognitive Therapy for Depression.* New York: Guilford Press.

Shantideva, Wallace, V. and Wallace, B. (1977). *A Guide to the Bodhisattva Way of Life.* Ithaca, New York: Snow Lion Publications.

Siegel, D., (2010b). *The Mindful Therapist: A Clinician's Guide to Mindsight and Neural Integration.* New York: W.W. Norton & Company.

Siegel, D. (2010a). *Mindsight: The New Science of Personal Transformation.* New York: Bantam.

Silverman, E.-M. (2012). Why Seek Therapy. Paper presented at the 15th Annual ISAD Online Conference, October.

Silverman, E.-M. (2011). What to Expect from Mindfulness. Paper presented at the 14th annual ISAD Online Conference, October.

Silverman, E.-M. (2010). My Stuttering is Me. Paper presented at the 13th Annual ISAD Online Conference, October.

Silverman, E.-M. (2009c). "Learning to Sit," 175-179. In E.-M. Silverman, *Mind Matters: Setting the Stage for Satisfying*

Clinical Service. A Personal Essay. Charleston: BookSurge Publishing.

Silverman, E.-M. (2009b). Doing The Work. Paper presented at the 12th Annual ISAD Online Conference, October.

Silverman, E.-M. (2009a). *Mind Matters: Setting the Stage for Satisfying Clinical Service. A Personal Essay.* Charleston, South Carolina: BookSurge Publishing.

Silverman, E.-M., (2008). Happily Every After. Paper Presented at the 11th Annual ISAD Online Conference.

Silverman, E.-M. (2007). Creating Conditions for Change. Paper Presented at the 10th Annual ISAD Online Conference

Silverman, E.-M., (2006b). Mind Matters. 9th Annual ISAD Online Conference, October.

Silverman, E.-M., (2006a). "A Personal Choice." *The ASHA Leader*, Vol. 11 (16), p. 47.

Silverman, E.-M. (2005), *Shenpa*, Stuttering, and Me. Paper presented at the 8th Annual ISAD Online Conference, October.

Silverman, E.-M. (2003). My Personal Experience with Stuttering and Meditation. Paper presented at the 6th Annual ISAD Online Conference, October.

Silverman, E.-M. (2001). *Jason's Secret.* Indianapolis: First Books.

Silverman, E.-M. (2000). *Jason's Secret:* What It Feels Like to Stutter. 3rd Annual International ISAD Online Conference, October.

Silverman, E.-M. (1986). A The Female Stutterer, 35-63. In K. St. Louis (Ed.), *The Atypical Stutterer*. New York: Academic Press.

Silverman, E.-M. (1973). Clustering: A characteristic of preschoolers' speech disfluency. *J. Speech Hearing Res.*, 16, 578-583.

Silverman, E.-M., and Williams, D. (1968). A comparison of stuttering and non-stuttering children in terms of five measures of oral language development. *J. Com. Dis.*, Vol. 1 (4), pp. 305-309.

Smalley, S. and Winston, D. (2010). *Fully Present: The Science, Art, and Practice of Mindfulness*. Cambridge, Massachusetts: Da Capo. Lifelong Books.

Steiner, C. (1994). *Scripts People Live. Transactional Analysis of Life Scripts*. New York: Grove Press.

Tolle, E. (2005). *The Power of Now*. London: Hodder & Staughton.

von Franz, M.-L. (1964). "The Process of Individuation," pp. 58-230. In C.G. Jung, (Ed.), *Man and His Symbols*. New York: Doubleday.

Weil, A. (1995). *Spontaneous Healing*. New York: Alfred A. Kopf.

Whitney, M. (1985). *Matter of Heart: The Extraordinary Journey of C. G. Jung Into the Soul of Man*. New York: Kino International Corporation. (DVD)

Willard, C. (2010). *Child's Mind. How Mindfulness Can Help Our Children Be More Calm, Focused, and Relaxed*. Berkeley, California: Parallax Press

Williams, D. (2004). *The Genius of Dean Williams*. Memphis, Tennessee: The Stuttering Foundation of America.

Williams, D.E. (1957). "A point of view about 'stuttering.'" *Journal of Speech & Hearing Disorders, 22*, 3, 390-397.

Winston, D. (2010). "Saying yes to an open heart." *Buddhadarmha: The Practitioner's Quarterly*, Summer, 31- 32.

Woollums, S. and Brown, M. (1979). *TA: The Total Handbook of Transactional Analysis*. Englewood Cliffs, N.J.: Prentice-Hall, Inc.

Resources

Websites

Mindfulness Meditation

Insight Meditation Society, http://www.dharma.org (on-site instruction)

Spirit Rock Meditation Center, http://www.spiritrock.org (on-site instruction)

Inquiring Mind, http://www.inquiringmind.com (resource guide for local Instruction)

The UCLA Institute Mindfulness Awareness Research Center, http://marc.ucla.edu/ (mindfulness meditation classes on site and online)

Mindful, http://www.mindful.org (mindfulness-based approaches to issues of daily life)

Mindfulness and Neuroscience Research

Center for Investigating Healthy Minds, www.investigatinghealthyminds.org (multidisciplinary research into healthy qualities of states and their effect on the body and the brain)

Mind & Life Institute, www.MindandLife.org (an international organization devoted to scientific study of the mind, i.e., contemplative science)

Stuttering Problems and Stuttering Help

European League of Stuttering Associations, http://www.stuttering.ws

International Stuttering Association, http://www.isastutter.org (information)

Israel Stuttering Association, http://www.ambi.org.il

The American Speech-Language-Hearing Association, http://www.asha.org (national credentialing body for speech-language pathologists includes information for the public including a therapist locator link)

The British Stammering Association, http://www.stammering.org (information and products)

The Indian Stammering Association, http://www.stammering.in (information, discussion forums)

The National Stuttering Association, http://nsastutter.org (information, products, and conferences)

The Stuttering Foundation, http://www.stutteringhelp.org (information and products for caregivers, professionals, and employers including a therapist locator)

The Stuttering Homepage, http://www.mnsu.edu/comdis/kuster/(information, portal to ISAD, International Stuttering Awareness Day Conferences, and archive of conference presentations)

Books

Mindfulness

Salzberg, S. (2011). *Real Happiness. The Power of Mindfulness. A 28 Day Program.* New York: Workman Books.

Chödrön, P. (2010). *Taking the Leap. Freeing Ourselves from Old Habits and Fears.* Boston: Shambhala Publications.

Hahn, T.N. (2002). *Be Free Where You Are.* Berkeley, California: Parallax Press.

Kabat-Zinn, J. (2005). *Coming to Our Senses. Healing Ourselves and The World Through Mindfulness.* New York: Hyperion.

Kornfield, J. (2009). *The Wise Heart. A Guide to the Universal Teachings of Buddhist Psychology.* New York: Bantam.

Stuttering

Guitar, B., (2005). *Stuttering: An Integrated Approach to Its Nature and Treatment.* Baltimore: Lippincott Williams & Wilkins.

Silverman, E.-M. (2001). *Jason's Secret.* Indianapolis: First Books.

Magazines

Buddhadharma: The Practioners' Quarterly Buddhadharma Online: www.thebuddhadharma.com

Shambhala Sun Shambhala Sun Online: www.shambhalasun.com *Tricycle Magazine: The Buddhist Review*

Tricycle Magazine Online: www.tricycle.com

Audio and Visual Recordings

Brown, E. (2008). *How to Cook Your Life*. New York: Lionsgate. (An interview with an American Zen priest who also is a cook that includes a demonstration of walking meditation) (DVD)

Kornfield, J. (1996). *The Inner Art of Meditation*. Boulder, Colorado: Sounds True, Inc. (Introduction to forms of *shamatha-vipassana* sitting meditation) (VHS TAPE)

Phillips, J., Stein, A., and Kukura, A. (2010). *Dhamma Brothers*. Freedom Behind Bars. (A documentary depicting the teaching of vipassana during a 10-day retreat in a maximum security prison) (DVD)

Acknowledgements

This book reflects my understanding of mindfulness practice as taught by Sylvia Boorstein, Pema Chödrön, Thich Nhat Hanh, Dzigar Kongtrül, Jack Kornfeld, Sakyong Mipham, Sharon Salzberg, Jon Kabat-Zinn, and by H. H. The Dalai Lama. Practicing mindfulness has helped me grow ever stronger to meet life's challenges with increasing equanimity and to speak and communicate with growing ease and satisfaction.

The stories I have heard from and about people with stuttering problems learning to speak and to live with greater ease and the accounts I have heard and read from speech pathologists about their commitment to help people with stuttering problems have helped guide me to become a more skilled, compassionate person and therapist.

To them all, on behalf of those who may read this book, I offer my profound gratitude.

About The Author

Ellen-Marie Silverman, Ph.D., Fellow of the American Speech-Language-Hearing Association, was Director of the Fluency Clinic at Marquette University. She holds the Ph.D. in speech pathology from the University of Iowa, and was a post-doctoral fellow in developmental psycholinguistics at The University of Illinois, Urbana-Champaign. She later trained as a Transactional Analysis counselor. Dr Silverman, a speech pathologist for more than 40 years, has been a member of the faculties of The University of Illinois at Urbana-Champaign, Marquette University, and The Medical College of Wisconsin. More recently, she has been CEO of TSS, Inc., a healthcare staffing support service she founded.

Dr. Silverman has been practicing *shamatha-vipassana* mindfulness meditation since 1996. In 2003, she recognized that the Tibetan Buddhist concept of *shenpa*, the sense we all have of feeling hooked and our habituated desire to flee the experience, incisively described the development and persistence of her stuttering problem and those of clients she has known. Incorporating *shenpa* work into her *shamatha-vipassana* meditation practice along with the mindfulness practices of *maitri, lojong,* the recitation of *gathas,* and *tonglen* then applying these strategies to her stuttering problem has helped her speak with increasing ease, confidence, and satisfaction.

Dr. Silverman has presented nationally and internationally to colleagues and students about the nature, prevention, and treatment of stuttering problems. She has shared her experience applying mindfulness to stuttering at several International Stuttering Awareness Day Online Conferences for people who have stuttering problems and for professionals, students-in-training, and people interested in stuttering.

The recipient of research awards, Dr. Silverman has published extensively in peer-reviewed publications, contributed chapters to textbooks, and authored a textbook on clinical practice, *Mind Matters. Setting the Stage for Satisfying Clinical Service. A Personal Essay.* She wrote *Jason's Secret,* a novel for readers from 9 to 12, about a 10 year-old boy taking his first steps to constructively resolve his stuttering problem.

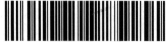